Nursing Competence

A guide to professional development

Edited by

Betty Kershaw

Edward Arnold
A division of Hodder & Stoughton
LONDON MELBOURNE AUCKLAND

© 1990 Betty Kershaw

First published in Great Britain 1990

British Library Cataloguing in Publication Data

Nursing competence.
1. Great Britain. Nurses. Professional education
I. Kershaw, Betty
610.73071141

ISBN 0-340-51841-3

Whilst the advice and information in this book is believed to be true
and accurate at the date of going to press, neither the author nor
the publisher can accept any legal responsibility or liability for any
errors or omissions that may be made.

Typeset in 10/11pt California by Colset Pte. Ltd., Singapore
Printed and bound in Great Britain for Edward Arnold, the
educational academic and medical division of Hodder and
Stoughton Limited, Mill Road, Dunton Green, Sevenoaks, Kent
TN13 2YA by Richard Clay Ltd, Bungay, Suffolk

Contents

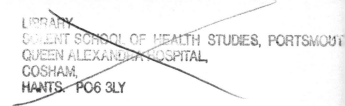
List of contributors

Maureen Eccleston **BA, RGN, DN, Cert.Ed**, is Head, School of Nursing and Health Studies, Stockport College of Further and Higher Education.

Marjorie Gott **BA, PhD, RGN, SCM, HV, RNT**, is Senior Lecturer and Post-Doctoral Nursing Research Fellow, Department of Health and Social Welfare, The Open University.

Mary Harrison **BA, MLS, ALA**, is Librarian, Stockport, Tameside and Glossop College of Nursing.

Margaret Johnston **RGN, DN, RCNT**, is Tutor, Enrolled Nurse Developments, Oxford Health Authority.

John Kelly **RGN, RMN, Dip.N, MIPM**, is Regional Nurse Education and Development Adviser, North West Regional Health Authority.

Reg Pyne **RGN**, is Director for Professional Conduct, The United Kingdom Central Council for Nursing, Midwifery and Health Visiting.

Nan Stalker **RGN, RCNT, RNT, ONC, BA, Dip.N**, is Senior Tutor, Continuing Education, Western College of Nursing and Midwifery, Glasgow.

Helena Stockford **BTEC(Hons), C.Biol, MA(Biol)**, is Principal, Mid-Warwickshire College of Further Education (formerly at South Manchester Community College).

Stephen G. Wright **RGN, DN, RCNT, DANS, RNT, MSc**, is Consultant Nurse, Nursing Development Unit, Tameside General Hospital.

Reg Pyne
Director for Professional Conduct
The United Kingdom Central Council for
Nursing, Midwifery and Health Visiting

Introduction
Professional responsibility

As I commence the writing of the first chapter of this book on 'Nursing Competence' I recall that, for a significant period of time in the 1970s, there regularly appeared in the national press and some journals and magazines an advertisement placed by the Department of Health and Social Security aimed at encouraging young people to train as nurses.

The words of that advertisement urged those who saw and read it to see the British State Registered Nurse (SRN) or Registered General Nurse (RGN) qualification as 'a passport to the world'. Those who were contemplating seeking entry to courses of nursing education in schools of nursing, lured by that advertisement, were even then being misled, since by the time it was appearing many countries had introduced very different arrangements for the education and training of nurses. Having done so they were (quite reasonably) measuring applications for registration from persons trained and registered outside their own territory against the content of their own professional education programmes and the demands made of students completing those programmes successfully.

One result of this change effected by nurse registration authorities in other countries was that, even while the 'passport to the world' theme was still being used as the focus of nurse training recruitment advertising, nurses newly emerging from training programmes were finding that the world apparently did not include some of the countries (notably all of North America) in which they most wanted to register, practice and obtain experience to serve them in good stead for their future.

At the same time some of their fellow British trained practitioners of longer standing in the profession also found themselves rejected when seeking to travel and practise nursing in other countries. One of the major reasons for this was that their training programmes (from several years' earlier) were deemed to compare even less favourably with those by then operating in the countries to which they were seeking to travel. A further reason (and, for the purposes of this book, a highly significant reason) was that this second group of would-be travellers were rarely able to demonstrate that they had taken any steps since initial registration to extend their knowledge, enhance their skills and question the basis of their professional practice. In other words, that which might have been regarded as bridging the gap and making such an applicant for registration acceptable (when not so regarded on a strict comparison of nursing education programmes) did not exist either at all or in identifiable documentary form.

It would seem that the mythology promulgated by that 'passport to the world' advertisement was very powerful. It was also clear that it had much to answer for.

It would be unreasonable, however, to attach excessive blame to those who designed and placed the advertisement. Their main aim was to try to ensure the existence of a professional nursing workforce to meet the needs of the United Kingdom, even though they were using the idea of world travel as a selling point. Some blame must attach to them, however, since, rather than use their position of influence and power to destroy a myth, they acted to perpetuate it. To publish a statement which implied that 'British is Best' was both consistent with and underlined the complacent attitude towards continuing education and the need to maintain and update competence that has hampered and still hampers British nursing. The profession itself has been responsible for the creation and perpetuation of a philosophy for nursing which has placed very little value on maintaining competence.

If you are tempted to the view that I am overstating my case I suggest that you would not draw such a conclusion if, like me, your professional employment had required you to sit for a number of years with the Disciplinary Committee (of the former General Nursing Council for England and Wales) and the Professional Conduct Committee (of the United Kingdom Central Council for Nursing, Midwifery and Health Visiting) as their respective members considered whether the practitioners appearing before them should lose or retain the right to practise in their profession.

Time after time it has become clear that the respondent practitioner before the committee is yet another one of those so deluded as to believe that, on the day that registration was first achieved, he or she was equipped for all of the world and for all time, with no need to open the textbooks again, no need to read professional journals, no need to engage in intelligent conversation with professional colleagues and certainly no need to engage in any further form of study. But also, time after time, it has become clear that it is that individual's failure to do exactly those things and consequent failure to maintain and develop competence that has led him or her to become involved in the kind of incident or develop that pattern of behaviour which results in complaints which place his or her registration status in jeopardy.

That is all by way of asserting (if you require such an incentive) that there is a powerful enlightened self-interest argument for maintaining your competence. Since you have chosen to read this book I take it that you have no desire to practise in the kind of defensive manner that would be consistent with that enlightened self-interest approach. It is much more likely that you are a practitioner who recognises and respects the primacy of the patient's interests and that, in consequence, you wish to take such measures and do such things as will best serve those interests. It is probable that, in so doing, you may well enhance both the level of satisfaction that you derive from your professional practice and your career progression.

It seems clear that those people (both within the nursing profession or supporting from outside its desire to progress) who strove successfully to influence the wording of the Nurses, Midwives and Health Visitors Act of 1979 to include the requirement that standards of training and professional conduct be improved and to refer to further training for the first time in primary legislation had recognised the need for a change in both emphasis and direction.

What is certain is that, from the very day (1 July 1983) on which that Act came fully into operation and it succeeded to the regulatory and registration function of the former statutory bodies for nursing, midwifery and health visiting, the United Kingdom Central Council for Nursing, Midwifery and Health Visiting (UKCC) has sought to emphasise that the exercise of personal professional accountability requires that practitioners maintain and improve their knowledge and competence, not as a matter of personal or professional self-aggrandisement, but in order that the interests of the public and of patients and clients be satisfactorily met.

The Council's principal instrument for achieving the required change of attitude and level of understanding has been the Code of Professional Conduct for the Nurse, Midwife and Health Visitor. Both the first edition of this important document (issued July 1983) and the second/current edition (issued November 1984) have included clauses which set out the Council's expectations of the people on its register in unequivocal terms.

It is perhaps unfortunate, though to some degree understandable, that many practitioners, when opening this important document, leap to the point numbered '1' and fail to read the introductory paragraphs out of which not only that clause but all the numbered clauses grow. I suggest that, on each and every occasion that any person on the register either reads or cites such a clause in a document sent to another person (e.g. their manager), those introductory paragraphs should also be read or quoted.

I hold and express this view for the simple reason that the first introductory paragraph makes it clear that the form of conduct required of persons on its register by the UKCC, and laid out for public view in the Code, is that which will serve the interests of the public in general terms, and particularly when they are cast in the role of patients or clients of nurses. Let me remind you or inform you that the introductory paragraph states:

> Each registered nurse, midwife and health visitor shall act, at all times, in such a manner as to justify public trust and confidence, to uphold and enhance the good standing and reputation of the profession, to serve the interest of society, and above all to safeguard the interests of individual patients and clients.

The purpose of the form of conduct described having been stated, the next paragraph provides the stem out of which all the numbered paragraphs of the Code grow. This states:

> Each registered nurse, midwife and health visitor is accountable for his or her practice, and, in the exercise of professional accountability shall . . .

From these few but extremely important words it can be seen that the various factors contained within the 14 clauses that follow are matters for which the individual practitioner bears a personal professional accountability. In other words, he or she may be called to account for any failure to meet the requirements stated and thus to fail to be the kind of practitioner portrayed in the opening paragraph.

In this context it is important to note that the UKCC, having given practitioners advice as to what it expects of them, now uses exactly that advice as the backcloth against which to consider complaints alleging misconduct in a professional sense against individual practitioners. Phrases from within the introductory paragraph (above) feature frequently within charges before the Professional Conduct Committee, as also does the whole of certain of the numbered clauses. The difference is that they are preceded by words to the effect that the practitioner is guilty of misconduct for his or her failure to do as the quoted clause requires.

The message emerging from the Code of Professional Conduct to be applied to the subject of maintaining competence therefore seems clear. You — not someone else acting on your behalf or whose instructions you may have followed — can be called to account for what you decide to do, for what you fail to do and for matters occurring within your sphere of influence. In other words, these are matters at the very heart of our professional responsibility. The Code is a document, the words of which are no sinecure. It is a document which you ignore only at your peril. It is a document which, together with those key clauses of the Nurses, Midwives and Health Visitors Act out of which it grows, states both the importance of and the case for maintaining competence. In so doing it surely helps to make the case for the existence and development of the wide range of further educational opportunities which are explained by the authors of several of the chapters of this book.

It is assumed that only two clauses in the Code of Professional Conduct have a bearing upon the subject of our competence as practitioners, these being those numbered '3' and '4'. Linked with their stem sentence, these read:

> Each registered nurse, midwife and health visitor is accountable for his or her practice, and, in the exercise of professional accountability shall:
>
> Take every reasonable opportunity to maintain and improve professional knowledge and competence.
>
> Acknowledge any limitations of competence and refuse in such cases to accept delegated functions without first having received instruction in regard to those functions and having been assessed as competent.

It is true, of course, that these two clauses relate to the subject of maintaining competence in a direct and obvious way.

In some ways to set them down at all is to state the obvious. It was necessary to do so, however, because only a small minority of practitioners seem to avail themselves of the opportunities provided by their employers and professional organisations and fewer still go beyond such provision and take steps on their own initiative. Clause 3 of the Code both was and is necessary as a statement to each practitioner.

So also was and is clause 4. It is a matter of serious concern that so many people within the profession fail to recognise the degree and nature of their own vulnerability, fail to acknowledge that there are limitations to their competence, and blithely accept instructions to perform a task or administer a substance when they do not have the knowledge to be sure that it is reasonable in the circumstances.

Conduct of this kind often places patients at risk and sometimes causes irrevocable damage. The damage to the practitioner's personal and professional life can also be considerable.

It is my contention, however, that all the other clauses of the Code relate to that aspect of an individual practitioner's professional responsibility that is concerned with maintaining competence. For example, clause 12 requires that the practitioner, in the context of his or her knowledge and experience and sphere of authority, assists peers and subordinates to develop professional competence in accordance with their needs. This simply cannot be done by those within the profession who have not maintained and improved their own competence. Therefore failure to maintain your own competence means that you fail your patients both directly and indirectly.

The terms of clause 6 of the Code presuppose that, in a society shared by persons of various ethnic origins, practitioners will see it as essential that they have sufficient knowledge about the customs, values and beliefs of their fellow citizens and a sufficiently open and inquiring approach to their own practice to make its expectation achievable. Perhaps this is a reminder for us that some of the additional knowledge we require, and indeed some of the new sensitivities we need to develop, though of importance to us in our professional practice, might need to be acquired through channels that are not part of the normally accepted professional further education process.

As for the other clauses, I suggest the following for your consideration.

- *Re* Clause 1, you cannot promote and safeguard the well-being and interests of patients/clients if you are not professionally competent to meet the needs of the present time as distinct from the needs of whatever year in which you became registered.
- *Re* Clause 5, you cannot work in a truly collaborative and co-operative manner with other health care professionals unless you are sufficiently informed to discuss the needs of patients/clients as a full member of a caring team and from a sound knowledge base.
- *Re* Clause 7, 8 and 9 (concerned with conscientious objection, privileged access and confidentiality), you cannot arrive at judgements that are your own, appropriate in the circumstances and able to be justified, unless you have first become clear about the ethical concepts that underlie these parts of the Code.
- *Re* Clauses 10 and 11 (concerned with the environment of care and the workload and pressures on colleagues), your prospects of making articulate representations in a form that is likely to have impact will be enhanced if some consideration of methods of com-

munication has featured in some part of your continuing education.

In summary, I am arguing that the Code of Professional Conduct in its entirety is something of a clarion call to maintain competence. Failure to do all in your power to maintain your competence might well be construed as a betrayal of those people called patients and clients who, when at their most frightened, vulnerable and dependent, place themselves into the care of those they know to possess qualifications in nursing.

Earlier in this chapter I described the Code of Professional Conduct as the UKCC's principal means of seeking to achieve the change in attitude and understanding that is required. It has not been the only means adopted. The promotion of a new approach to education in preparation for registration, the fruits of which are now beginning to be seen, has stimulated a great deal of exciting new thinking about the purpose of professional education. The first of the new style programmes now being in operation, the UKCC has turned its attention to the equally important question of education beyond registration. Even as this book has been in preparation, a new UKCC project (the Post-Registration Education and Practice Project) has been launched. The initial information released about this project indicates the application of a framework that first considers the nature of professional practice, moves on to consideration of the processes of professional education and development, all as a means of drawing some conclusions about the requirements for continuing competence to practice. I hope that you will agree that this demonstrates the UKCC's determination to respond to the challenges and grasp the opportunities provided by the Nurses, Midwives and Health Visitors Act of 1979. It is essential that large numbers of people within the profession match that determination by, of their own volition rather than compulsion, grasping the opportunities that exist, campaigning for an extension of opportunities and persuading the doubters and cynics that the maintenance of competence is essential to competent practice.

I think that we should be in no doubt that this is part of a positive professional revolution. It now seems clear that to be compliant and submissive, and to respond to the instructions of others in an unthinking, unquestioning way has been to act in a manner that does not best serve the interests of patients.

Those interests are better served by practitioners who are honest, open, questioning and challenging in their approach to the delivery of care. Those qualities link directly with the maintenance of competence. It is a matter of professional responsibility to develop and nurture those qualities.

I have been afforded the opportunity, prior to writing this chapter, to read the text that follows. I have found it very informative and extremely challenging. Clearly there have been a significant number of people in the profession who have been demanding continuing education. It is my earnest hope that this book will not only assist them to formulate their demands but will convince many more that fulfilment of their professional responsibility should involve them in becoming similarly persistent and provide them with a useful information base from which to operate.

Helena Stockford
Principal
Mid-Warwickshire College of Further Education

1 What further education has to offer

Introduction

Perhaps to a greater extent than in any other sector of the education system, further education (FE) has always felt the need to provide flexible learning opportunities for students. As every lecturer and manager in FE knows, there has never been any guarantee that students will enrol on programmes of study in FE, or that employers will co-operate in providing training opportunities for their staff through their local FE college. In order to continue to survive and prosper against a background of decline in apprentice training, alternative training opportunities provided by employers in the workplace, continual changes in funding mechanisms and levels, and the need to respond to an ever shifting pattern of training requirements and demography, FE has always needed to market itself energetically and to ensure that once students enrol on programmes of study they stay there until their studies have been successfully completed. There are other reasons too why provision is particularly and increasingly student-centred. For many, FE, or continuing education as it is frequently labelled, represents a 'second chance' to climb the rungs of the ladder leading to professional careers or to update skills and knowledge before transferring from one career route or level to another. Compared to the time students spend in the other sectors of education, they tend not to stay in FE for very long. Therefore, the time in FE needs to be spent wisely and to maximum effect in filling and bridging knowledge gaps and 'topping up' prior learning, whether this has been gained formally in a structured learning environment or experientially. For all these reasons a 'good' college of further education is continually seeking to design courses which meet its current users' learning needs and, in so doing, expend a great deal of effort identifying those needs and using them as a basis for an individual learning programme. Gone are the days of many of the 'off the peg' courses which started in September, ran from 9.00 a.m.–4.00 p.m. each day of every week for one or two academic years, and finished with a formal end examination. Replacing them are modular and often branching learning programmes whose constituent parts can each lead to the award of some form of accreditation, which is cumulative, as the programme progresses. Students can follow these programmes through a variety of learning modes, ranging from regular attendance at set times to 'drop in' sessions at irregular intervals. Also the programmes can operate on a 'roll-on-roll-off' basis throughout an academic year, and much of the time that is spent in contact with tutors is used to develop skills such as study, numeracy, analytical and communication. The emphasis is placed on the acquisition and practice of these skills rather than in imparting factual knowledge on a 'chalk and talk' basis when this can be provided by a variety of other delivery mechanisms such as 'self instructing' print-based, tape and video materials. FE nowadays can be compared to one of those American service stations where the objective is not only to top up and fuel users' enthusiasm, but also to provide them with career route maps and, if necessary, wipe the windscreen so that they can see where they are going! The users' requirements are diagnosed, checked and specifically catered for when they 'drop in'; they do not stay for very long, and most of them progress further – even if sometimes this involes a 'U' turn or two along the way.

The demographic trends predicted to affect the nursing profession so drastically in the next few years are already affecting FE. Up until recently the largest traditional client group entered FE at 16. The decline in 16-year-old school leavers available to enter FE has been, to say the least, dramatic. In Manchester, for example, the number of 11 to 16-year-olds in county and Church of England high schools fell from 24 770 in 1980 to 16 707 in 1987 and is still on the decline. The number is unlikely to rise again significantly until 1995. However, it is a mark of FE's capacity to survive and respond that, despite this level of decline in 16-year-olds which is being experienced across the country, a record 1 745 000 students enrolled nationally for FE courses in the autumn of 1987 (Libby and Hill, 1988). This is because many colleges have already begun to focus more specifically on the huge number of adults who can presently benefit from continuing education and training. Having prepared people for work, FE can also 'update' people during their working lives. The Department of Education and Science's Professional, Industrial and Commercial Updating Programme (PICKUP) was devised in the early 1980s when it was evident that the number of 'updating' adults in work was low and actually declining. The PICKUP initiative for adults seeking retraining and updating has helped colleges to increase both the quantity and quality of training provided to employers on a full cost basis. Between 1985/6 and 1986/7 the number of students on updating courses in England, Wales and Scotland (Northern Ireland have a similar but separate initiative) increased by nearly 40 per cent. PICKUP's target is that one in ten of the working population in England should receive this kind of training by the early 1990s. Since the start of the PICKUP programme FE colleges have demonstrated their competence in delivering updating courses and have grasped the opportunities available to them. Staff are themselves being 'updated' on their teaching techniques and approaches in dealing with adult learners.

As long ago as 1982, the Advisory Council for Adult and Continuing Education defined the changes of teaching approach required in their report *Continuing Education – From Policies to Practice* as follows.

> Adults will still want to benefit from face to face tuition, but the teaching methods used in initial education are not always suitable for adults. Adult learners often bring to their learning a determination to succeed because they have deliberately chosen to study for a specific purpose. Because of their wider experience of life they are able to appreciate the relevance of their learning in ways not possible for younger students and they can generally take a much more active part in their own learning.
>
> They also face other problems which the young do not. Having spent time away from regular study, many adults are no longer familiar with the techniques of study and they may often require individual help to overcome these difficulties and acquire the necessary skills. Education needs to take account of these different strengths and weaknesses.

It is because of this recognition of the needs of adult learners together with 'user friendly' approaches in terms of flexibility that many nurses already enrol with colleges of FE to 'update' their skills. This is increasingly true for those nurses who have insufficient alternatives in terms of updating at work and through continuing education programmes in-house to provide the learning opportunities they require. We therefore consider it even more important that when nurses enrol we provide not only the learning programmes they need, but also the support mechanisms that go with them, and the type of non-threatening and personalised learning experiences that will ensure client satisfaction.

In considering the type and range of FE provision which is appropriate to the continuing educational needs of qualified nurses, it is firstly important to stress that in the majority of colleges the specific study programmes available provide only part of the total student service. This service begins when the student makes the first approach to the college. They may have been advised to do so at work, or they may be responding to some form of publicity produced by the college or careers service. Many students hear about FE provision from friends and colleagues who have studied in FE themselves at some time. By whatever means the information reaches the potential students, it is true to say that most of them possess only a rudimentary picture of what is involved, have more questions than answers, and in many cases really do not know whether the learning programmes as advertised will suit their requirements or not and to understand that access and open and distance learning courses allow flexibility of studying. They need to know for instance that an access course is an alternative entry route into further and/or higher education or professional training. It does not necessarily involve qualifications such as GCSE or A level and the method of delivery of the course is geared to the needs and prior learning experiences of mature students. Also that open learning is a method of individual study where the client/student can negotiate the whole process of learning including the time, the place, the length, the format and the range of course to be followed. Distance learning is a term used to describe a course of study where any kind of face-to-face tuition is impossible or extremely difficult.

Even more common are those adults who wish to return to some type of study, but who do not have any fixed ideas as to what subjects or levels of study they should undertake. This is hardly surprising because the first stage in any learning programme should be a 'diagnosis' of needs, present academic levels, and prior learning. This assessment is undertaken in college via an initial interview between the student and counsellor or course tutor. The result of the process should be a negotiated learning programme tailored to meet the student's individual requirements. Information should also be supplied to students about all the services provided in the college. For example, many nurses who work shifts are only free to pursue studies at times when their pre-school children cannot be looked after by their partner or relatives. A place booked in a college creche during these study periods can sometimes solve the problem for unemployed nurses. A college counsellor, there to advise on current Department of Social Services (DSS) regulations in relation to students' ability to attend college on a part-time basis, can relieve anxiety and inform the student how they can pursue their learning programmes without loss of benefit (currently known as the 'under 21 hour rule'). No matter how short the attendance period per week, or how irregular, the student services of the college should provide each individual student as far as possible with the support required to facilitate their learning processes.

Having described in general terms the type of provision and facilities available within FE today, no chapter on FE could be complete without outlining at least some of the specific learning programmes and modes of delivery on offer. This can best be illustrated by describing programmes provided at one large city college, South Manchester Community College, which offers a wide selection of courses to qualified nurses to assist them in maintaining competence. It does not purport to be a comprehensive survey, but to be an illustration of the type of provision likely to be available in any local FE institution. The learning opportunities available to qualified nurses within the College fall into five main categories.

- The students can 'infill' into specific modules or sections of existing learning programmes running during the day. For example, the College offers Business and Technician Education Council (BTEC) courses at National and First Level leading to professional training within the caring professions and containing, among others, units in Health Education, Psychology, Human Biology, Mathematics and Communications Skills. It is possible for qualified nurses to 'infill' into these classes in specific subject areas and obtain accreditation in the form of a BTEC Certificate of Achievement for completion of individual units. Several City and Guilds of London Institute qualifications are also offered which are modularised and can be undertaken on a part-time day and evening basis.

- The College offers a wide range of General Certificates of Secondary Education (GCSE) and A levels during the day and evening. Each subject can be taken individually or combined with others to provide a specific learning programme to meet the needs of the individual. Each subject comprises approximately five hours of class contact per week so a range of combinations of several A and GCSE levels can be studied while still complying with the current DSS rules regarding 'Under 21 hour' attendance at College.

- Qualified nurses can also attend a range of short courses specifically designed to meet their requirements. These are offered as a range of 'workshops', either during the day or evening, on specific topic areas selected from within a group of print-based, tape and video packages provided by the Open University, the Open College and other learning materials providers. Both the Continuing Nurse Education programmes produced by Barnet and Manchester Distance Learning Project and the Management in Nursing Series produced by the Distance Learning Centre of South Bank Polytechnic are on offer. There is also a range of short courses developed to meet local needs, for example Health and Care, Issues Related to Work in the Community, and courses for primary health care teams to develop strategies for corporate working. For many of these courses, accreditation is available through BTEC, the Open University or the Manchester Open College Federation.

- Perhaps the most 'popular' range of learning programmes on offer to qualified nurses are those available on an open learning basis. As a result of several initiatives in education and training in recent years, many FE colleges now offer a range of open or flexible learning programmes. At South Manchester Community College 1500 students currently follow open learning courses. Such programmes have enormous advantages for the practising nurse and offer flexibility in terms of:
  — start date
  — time of study
  — place of study
  — pace of study

  In addition the inherent flexibility of such courses means that each individual nurse's learning programme can be customised to ensure that his/her specific training needs are being fulfilled. Since good quality open learning material contains clear explanations of the subject matter, a nurse need not feel tied to a college-based tutor but may also use a colleague 'mentor' to assist him/her in working through the course. This can be another important factor in ensuring that the course is completely tailored to meet the nurse's needs.

  One further advantage in following an open learning course is that through the individualised nature of the programme the nurse is encouraged to gain independence in his/her studying and learning. Clearly this is in itself a vital skill which will benefit the learner on any subsequent course he/she chooses to follow – whether this be an open learning course or a more 'traditional' course.

  There are many different types of open learning courses available. A few of those most favoured by the many nurses who enrol are briefly outlined below.

Continuing nurse education programmes, based on the Barnet and Manchester open learning material, are a series of 30-hour study modules which cover a range of topics including:
— the management of learning
— interpersonal skills
— introducing immunology
— the nature of cancer
— nursing today
— measurement in nursing
— approaches to psychology
— aspects of social psychology
— individualised patient care

Each of the modules is presented in a lively, interactive, open learning format, engaging the learner in work-based activities as well as presenting self-assessment questions. South Manchester Community College and Central Manchester College are now offering a BTEC Continuing Education Certificate in Nursing Studies based on these modules. Within this qualification, each individual unit leads to the award of a BTEC Certificate of Achievement. Enrolled nurses can gain exemption of up to six weeks off a conversion course as a result of taking appropriate BTEC approved modules.

Flexistudy courses South Manchester Community College, in common with many other FE colleges, offers a range of GCSE and A level courses which can be followed on an open learning basis. This means that the nurse could obtain these 'national' qualifications while at work which might otherwise be impossible if he/she had to attend formal classes at set times each week. Flexistudy courses typically operate by linking the student to a tutor in college. The tutor then guides the student through the course using specially prepared open learning materials so that the student carries out most of his/her work at a time and place which suits him/her. Student and tutor then meet at a mutually convenient time, approximately once every three weeks, for a 30 minute tutorial in which they discuss any problems the student may have experienced; important points that have been covered; assignments which have been completed; and the next section of work which must be completed before they meet again.

The National Examinations Board for Supervisory Studies (NEBSS) offers a wide range of nationally recognised awards to supervisory managers. By studying an appropriate selection of open learning units in their Super Series, students obtain NEBSS Module Awards which in turn lead to the Certificate in Supervisory

Management. The Super Series contains modules under the headings of:
— principles and practice of supervision e.g. team leading and taking decisions
— technical aspects of supervision e.g. quality codes and managing time
— communication e.g. writing skills
— economic and financial aspects e.g. control via budgets
— industrial relations e.g. training sessions, health and safety
  These modules are particularly useful for nurses who are interested in gaining promotion to management positions, and for practising ward sisters and staff nurses.

• *The Open College* is a national approach to vocational skills training using open learning methodology. The Open College use television and radio broadcasts and students can obtain tutor support from a network of open access centres (most of which operate from colleges of further education, or from a national distance learning centre). The majority of Open College courses lead to nationally recognised qualifications and their range of courses is constantly expanding and includes modules on introductory study skills; business and management; information technology; and practical skills. Although none of the current modules are especially geared towards nurses, there are many modules which the practising nurse would find both stimulating and an aid to their daily work performance.

The English National Board for Nursing, Midwifery and Health Visiting (ENB) in its circular *Spectrum of Opportunities for Enrolled Nurses* 1988/67/RMHLV, published in December 1988, have recognised some programmes offered by FE colleges as useful 'prior learning' and have quantified them in terms of 'exemption time' against conversion courses which enrolled nurses may wish to undertake in order to register with the UKCC. Schools of nursing offering conversion courses and also courses such as the new ENB 902 'Return to Nursing' course are also being encouraged to utilise appropriate open learning materials as part of their provision, and FE colleges are providing staff development programmes and consultancies to the nurses on aspects of open learning methodology.

There are many more opportunities to 'update' for qualified nurses currently available in local FE colleges and staff may also be willing to provide updating programmes on an 'outreach' basis in the workplace by negotiation between the college and appropriate nurse managers. But, even more importantly, staff are continually on the 'look-out' for fresh ideas and avenues for curriculum development. So, if you have specific learning requirements which are currently not being met, do go and talk to your local FE college, not to discover whether your requirements 'fit in' with their present provision, but whether they can provide you with the 'tailor made' programme you require.

Useful addresses

Business and Technician Education
   Council
Head Office
Central House
Upper Woburn Place
London WC1

Distance Learning Centre
South Bank Polytechnic
Room 1D35
South Bank Technopark
90 London Road
London SE1 6LN

City and Guilds of London
   Institute
75 Portland Place
London W1

English National Board
Victory House
170 Tottenham Court Road
London W1P OHA

Continuing Nurse Education
Barnet College
Russell Lane
Whetstone
London N20 OAY

The Open University
Walton Hall
Milton Keynes
Buckinghamshire MK7 6AA

References

Advisory Council for Adult and Continuing Education (1982). *Continuing Education: From Policies to Practice*. ACACE, London.

English National Board (1988/67/RMHLV). *Spectrum of Opportunities for the Enrolled Nurse*. ENB, London.

Libby, D. and Hill, R. (1988). Series of Further Education Publications. Obtainable from 2 Orange Street, London WC2.

Nan Stalker
Senior Tutor
Continuing Education
Western College of Nursing and Midwifery

2 Professional development

Early in 1982 nurses in Scotland became aware of the Report of the working party, chaired by Margaret Auld, entitled *Continuing Education for the Nursing Profession in Scotland*. The remit of the group was two fold:

— to suggest a framework within which existing and proposed courses of continuing education could fit
— to make recommendations for rationalising courses in order to use resources as efficiently as possible.

In many ways this group was leading the way for the profession nationally. It is to be hoped that they are not disappointed with the way the profession has gone since the Report was published. Their framework can only be described as visionary, identifying the following reasons for organising post-registration education and training:

— to prepare nurses to meet the accelerating rate of development in nursing, medical and technological services
— to enable nurses, many of whom will experience service breaks, to return to work and function effectively
— to discourage nurses from undertaking a programme in a speciality in which they do not intend to practise
— to enable the profession to meet the health care demands of a better informed public

It would be impossible to summarise the whole Report in this chapter without devaluing the work, and a strong recommendation is made that those interested should look at this document or at least read the Summary of Proposals. The findings indicate that all nurses taking up new employment require an induction or orientation programme, that each nurse should be responsible for seeking continuing education, and that management should provide adequate

opportunities for continuing education for all staff following registration. There should be provision for continuing education at
differing levels which could be provided initially by colleges/schools
of nursing and midwifery and later, as one progressed, by colleges of
further and higher education. The need for diplomas and degrees to
be available to the nurse was identified and links with outside
agencies (agencies within the academic world) were encouraged.

What happened to this Report? In a profession where some reports
have gathered dust on a shelf, it was hoped by many that it would not
happen to this Report. Around the same time as the Report was
published all General Nursing Councils were handing over to the new
National Boards, and the National Board for Nursing, Midwifery and
Health Visiting for Scotland (NBS) agreed in May 1983 with the
recommendation of the Report in principle. Elsewhere in the UK the
Report was debated; only the Welsh National Board have, as yet,
taken any formal action.

The first NBS reached implementation of the Report in March
1984. A definition of continuing education was quickly identified; a
definition that was borrowed from America and used in the original
Report.

> Continuing education in nursing consists of planned learning
> experiences beyond a basic nursing educational programme.
> These experiences are designed to promote the development of
> knowledge, skills, and abilities for the enhancement of nursing
> practice, thus improving health care to the public.
>
> (American Nurses Association, 1975)

The task assumed by the NBS was not an easy one as the course had
to meet the needs of all the newly-qualified nurses on all parts of the
United Kingdom Central Council Professional Register including
experienced nurses who had been unable as yet to benefit from
continuing education for whatever reason. A starting point had to be
identified for some stages of the programme and this is discussed later
in the chapter.

Before looking at the proposals, one very important matter should
be considered: Who will pay for continuing education? It was
previously assumed that management should provide continuing
education and indeed it is the local Health Boards who provide all
monitoring, human and material resources. This, of course, allows
for a variety of responses, some areas being better catered for than
others. However, the enthusiasm of the profession as a whole ensures
that the best possible use is made of any available resources. Perhaps
in the future the financial commitment will be the responsibility of

the NBS as with all other areas of nursing education, thus allowing for a more even distribution of available resources.

What were the proposals of the Post-Basic Committee formed by the NBS in 1984? They started with the newly-registered nurse and identified the need for a short orientation programme which could be common for all experienced nurses commencing a new post. This programme would be designed by each individual hospital and would meet local needs and local policies would be discussed and other administrative procedures identified; the total programme need not be more than 15 to 20 hours in length. One might well say 'What is new?' while others would be pleased to see such a recommendation. Following the orientation programme it was thought that a six month period of consolidation/induction would be beneficial to the newly-registered nurse with approximately 50 hours of theory, later to be reduced to 30 hours, included in the six months. Once again, the programme was left to local in-service education departments to design. These recommendations were made to the profession as early as July 1983, and Health Boards were encouraged to make some provision as early as possible to prevent a backlog of potential participants. As these initial programmes were to be designed locally and the NBS did not need to be notified as to the content, and indeed no valuation of the programme by the NBS was given, some Health Boards initiated programmes, others did not.

The next move by the NBS was perhaps the most exciting, especially to those involved in any way in continuing education either as a teacher or a participant. A small working group of the Post-Basic Committee was formed in March 1984 to look at what the original Report had called Clinical Studies 1, 2 and 3, but what the NBS preferred to call Professional Studies. The working group were given the following remit:

— to define the outcome(s) for those undertaking the courses
— to consider the methods by which students could study for the courses
— to consider the academic valuation of the courses, particularly in relation to the transferability of credits or other awards

Initially, and at the time of writing, two levels were identified; Professional Studies 1 and 2. The nurses who successfully completed level 2 would be potential charge nurses. The profession was to receive the deliberations of the working group as 'Guidelines for Continuing Education Professional Studies 1 and 2' in February 1985 and work commenced immediately in some colleges of nursing and midwifery to implement the new programme.

Professional Studies 1 was designed with the first level registered nurse who commenced training in 1982 as the principal client. This date was chosen as it was the start of a modular system of basic nurse education throughout Scotland. It is important to add that, although this date was identified, no first level registered nurse is excluded or exempt from the programme, although many nurse managers do give priority to modular-trained nurses. The programme consists of three modules (two of which are compulsory), each of nine weeks in length, which need not be taken consecutively or within any set period of time. The modules are intended to be generic in nature. Two of the module titles were identified by the working group: 'Interpersonal Relationships' and 'Learning, Teaching and Counselling'. Many exciting nursing modules are now available, such as 'Decision Making in the Health Service', 'Control of Aggression', 'Standards of Care' to name a few. The nurse would undertake the two compulsory modules and would select a third module according to his/her professional needs. These modules were devised by the colleges of nursing and midwifery in consultation with their clinical colleagues.

The colleges of nursing and midwifery were given very few restrictions in curriculum design, each module had to have ten days (60 hours) of theoretical content, and student-centred learning was encouraged as were (and is) flexible learning packages (see p. 6). Examinations were not stipulated, indeed most modules are designed without them, although some form of written assessment does take place. A committee was set up to look at each module submission document in great detail and NBS retains very tight control of national standards in relation to validating each module.

The nurse remains within the clinical area of employment for the clinical experience and there can be either day or night duty or rotation. On successful completion of each module, the nurse receives a Statement of Completion from the college of nursing and midwifery which is supplied by the NBS. After receiving three Statements, the nurse sends them to the NBS and receives a Professional Studies 1 Credit. Exemption can be received from either or both of the two stated modules by providing evidence of other study equating to content and time. Two accreditations are the limit.

The modules for Professional Studies 2, the next level in the programme of continuing education, are specific in nature. As elsewhere within the United Kingdom, Scotland had had for some time 52-week courses in a variety of specialities and the profession was advised to run out their programmes and look to the new guidelines. This now gave an opportunity to look afresh at the needs of the profession and design modules to meet new demands.

A similar format as for Professional Studies 1 was advised for Professional Studies 2. In order to receive a Credit three modules would have to be successfully completed. Each module would be a minimum of nine weeks, no maximum was laid down. It was expected that a nine-week module would have a 60 hour theoretical component, but should the module be longer the theoretical content would be altered accordingly. As with the Professional Studies 1 modules, there were no rules and regulations made about how one undertook modules and no time limit was set for the completion of the total programme if that was what the student wanted.

The NBS has a different system of validating the second level modules. A module submitted by a college of nursing and midwifery is initially read by the Professional Adviser in Continuing Education who could, if required, contact the college concerning any omissions. The submission is then passed to a specialist panel, usually composed of an equal number of nurse educationalists and clinical nurses currently active within the speciality. This group will spend time examining the submission document and liaising with the college of nursing and midwifery and relevant clinical areas until they are happy with the content. Following this, the Professional Adviser, along with a nurse educationalist and a clinical nurse, will visit all clinical areas proposed for use in the submission. This visit allows for discussion with service colleagues concerning the objectives, learning outcomes, assessment and evaluation and, indeed, the expectations of the nurse at the end of the module. Care is taken that no clinical area is overloaded with students at whatever stage in their career, and that the quality of patient care is of prime importance. The small visiting group then reports back to the specialist panel and, once everyone is satisfied about the standard and value of the module, recommendation for approval is made to the NBS itself, usually for a period of two to five years. This validating procedure can take some time, but it is the responsibility of the NBS to maintain standards of practice.

At this point it may be useful to compare the two levels of Professional Studies from an administrative point of view. Professional Studies 1 has three modules of nine weeks each, the submission is approved according to the document presented, and the number of participants for the module is indicated by the college of nursing and midwifery. The number of participants can vary between ten and 50 and all clinical areas can be used for experience. Professional Studies 2 also has three modules before a Credit is awarded. However, each module has to be a minimum of nine weeks. The number of participants is confirmed by the specialist panel according to the educational experiences available in the areas which receive approval, this therefore limits placements and the number participating may be between six and 20.

At present, fewer nurses will be able to complete Professional Studies 2 modules. However, more and more modules are being designed and in the future the nurse will have a wider choice.

How does the first level registered nurse make this decision? As most nurses are seconded to the module(s) by their employing authority, they usually select modules following a discussion with their nurse managers. An annual professional assessment or performance review can be most useful in assisting choice. Thus the choice of module(s) is made according to the area in which the nurse is employed; this not only assists in the career prospects of the individual, but improves the standards of patient care. Secondment itself has advantages: if only one module is available in a specific subject which is pertinent to the nurse, then the nurse does not need to resign to undertake this short module of perhaps nine or 12 weeks. The nurse also does not have the additional worry of seeking new employment which might distract from the educational experiences. As colleges of nursing and midwifery offer more Professional Studies 2 modules, the calendar of dates for modules will become more and more complex and a nurse may well find six months between modules pertinent to his/her needs, should more than one module be required.

What has the Professional Studies programme to offer the first level registered nurse? He/she can undertake the complete programme (three Professional Studies 1 modules) thus being awarded a Professional Studies 1 Credit, and three Professional Studies 2 modules, thus being awarded a Professional Studies 2 Credit. These two Credits can then be exchanged for a Diploma in Professional Studies awarded by the NBS and recordable with the United Kingdom Central Council Professional Register. However, the nurse may decide to only complete Professional Studies 1 or, indeed, if there is a pertinent module at Professional Studies 2 level which would enhance the nursing care in his/her present job, only undertake that module. Should the nurse change to a new job within another speciality, perhaps five years' later, then other module(s) may be taken.

No longer does a nurse commence a 52-week course in orthopaedic nursing and use only about two weeks of the theory and ten weeks of the clinical experience during the remainder of his/her working life. Now the nurse looks at the job he or she is doing and selects the appropriate modules.

For example, the nurse in an intensive care unit can select a module concerned with nursing the patient requiring ventilation, a second concerned with orthopaedic trauma nursing, and a third concerned with the patient undergoing haemodialysis. Another nurse in a similar unit might say that little haemodialysis is used in his/her unit and would replace this module with something in cardiovascular nursing. The nurse in an ophthalmic ward might select a module concerned with ophthalmic nursing, one on care of the elderly, and one related to nursing a person with diabetes. Hopefully the limit of options will be infinite and, indeed, modules will go out of vogue through time and be replaced by others.

The programme as discussed in this chapter has been offered in some colleges of nursing and midwifery throughout Scotland for enough time to be able to say that it is meeting the needs of the profession and, indeed, up to a point, is in line with the work identified by the Working Party on Continuing Education and Professional Development for Nurses, Midwives and Health Visitors. A third level is now required, possibly to be called Professional Studies 3.

What is developing in other countries in the United Kingdom

All three countries in the United Kingdom are currently planning programmes which credit previous learning. Wales is committed to the Certificate in Professional Practice which will be modular and open to both first and second level nurses. Northern Ireland has consulted with the profession and is aiming to announce a new scheme at the end of 1989. England, through the work of the ENB, is already reviewing continuing education courses and plans to announce its decisions early in 1990.

All in all, the Boards are aiming to reduce the time nurses spend repeating course work, by crediting and recognising previous learning. Where Scotland has led the others will surely follow, not necessarily with the same model but with similar models that are prepared to meet the needs of the nurses for whom they are responsible.

Useful addresses

National Board for Scotland
22 Queen Street
Edinburgh EH2 1JX

United Kingdom Central Council
  for Nursing, Midwifery and
  Health Visiting
23 Portland Place
London W1N 3AF

References

Continuing Education for the Nursing Profession in Scotland. A Report of a Working Party on Continuing Education and Professional Development for Nurses, Midwives and Health Visitors (1981). Available from the Library, Scottish Home and Health Department, New St Andrew's House, Edinburgh.

National Board for Nursing, Midwifery and Health Visiting for Scotland (1985). *Guidelines for Continuing Education: Professional Studies 1 and 2*. NBS, Edinburgh.

Wells, J. (1989). *The Directory of Continuing Education and Training for* Nurses. Newpoint, London.

Marjorie Gott
Senior Lecturer
Department of Health and Social Welfare
The Open University

3 The role of the Open University

There is currently wide and growing interest in continuing education for members of the nursing profession and the use of distance or open learning (see p. 6) as a means of providing this education.

There are a number of reasons for these trends. Foremost amongst these are the changes in the profession itself. Most nurses now know about the United Kingdom Central Council for Nursing, Midwifery and Health Visiting's (UKCC) intention to require nurses to provide evidence of having undertaken some form of continuing education when they re-register their intention to practice again. As the majority of nurses work full time, and a large proportion work unsociable hours, open learning is an uniquely attractive form of provision to nurses and to managers alike. Its main attraction is that it can be studied by anyone (there are no entry requirements), at any time, and in any place. It is therefore highly cost-effective. The open learning material is provided in a package and, depending upon the type and level of course studied, learning can be entirely independent, or students may be required to come together in groups from time to time. For Open University courses that have a group work element, a tutor is either provided by the Open University (certificated courses) or a group teaching pack is provided. This is generally used by the 'in house' staff trainer, manager, or staff group leader.

Other reasons for the growth of both continuing education and open learning in nursing are to do with planned major changes in basic and post basic nurse education (Project 2000 and Post Registration Education Practice Project (PREPP) – see Chapter 6) and changes in the health sector generally. These include the need to respond to major health problems (e.g. coronary heart disease, drug use) and demographic trends such as an increase in the ageing population. The scale of the educative task is so great, and the number of nurses to reach so large, that distance learning is now seen as a major form of provision. A good example of the potential of an open learning course to quickly and cheaply educate a large sector of the nursing workforce is provided by take up of the Open University course 'A Systematic Approach to Nursing Care'. This course was provided, with the support and approval of the Department of Health and Social Security and the Statutory Bodies in nurse education, to train nurses in a newly agreed standard method of nursing care, the nursing process, to be implemented throughout the United Kingdom (UK). To date, over 50 000 learning packages have been sold, many more will have studied the course because of multiple usage.

Open University courses normally have a five year life after which they may be updated or remade. 'A Systematic Approach To Nursing Care' is now being updated in line with professional needs and developments and an updating supplement is being written, selected readings provided, and an assessment package added. The new course will be available at the end of 1989 and a full Supplementary Package will be available as a separate item to update previous users of the course. Rewriting has brought the course up to 100 study hours in total and this gives it recognition as a significant study unit both within and outside the Open University. Within, the course can be assessed for credit; in other programmes it can either be a freestanding continuing education course, or part of qualifying training. The course is likely to be of considerable value in assisting those wishing to convert from enrolled nurse (EN) to registered general nurse (RGN) qualification (see Chapter 7).

Distance learning and open learning

Whilst many nurses may use learning packages at a distance, or study on their own, more and more are studying them as some part of professional or 'in house' training. This fairly new and unorthodox method of teaching is therefore increasingly being incorporated in traditional teaching provision where part or all of a package may be used. Examples of this kind of use can be found in district nurse, practice nurse, health visitor and general practitioner education and involves use of 'education for health' packages, such as 'Coronary Heart Disease; Reducing the Risk', 'Drug Use and Misuse' and 'Mental Health Problems in Old Age'. These three topics address current UK health priority and problem areas and both students in training and practitioners in the field need to know the type of nursing intervention that is required.

The use of packs in traditional training is why, increasingly, people talk about 'open', rather than 'distance' learning. Open implies that it can be used in any way, in any setting, not necessarily limited to distance (see p. 4).

Courses and learning packages

The attractiveness of a ready-prepared teaching package for those carrying training and educative responsibilities may appear obvious, but there can be drawbacks too; perhaps to do with occupational or institutional relevance. Design of course materials at the Open University takes these factors into account. Depending on the course followed, a learning pack will generally contain a course text (workbook with activities), a course reader (edited existing and newly-commissioned important readings), and a cassette (examples of practice, patients and nurses views). Group leader or teacher packs contain all of these and a teaching videotape and full set of notes linked to the materials in the individual student pack.

In designing the course a number of people come together and a number of common stages are gone through. Experts in the field to be studied write the text and advise on articles and audio and video material. Open University staff then transform the text into open learning style (make it user friendly!) and it is then sent out to potential students and other experts to work through and comment on. Following this, the final drafts are written and edits done. As a result of this extensive and expensive process of developmentally testing materials, professionally sound and occupationally relevant courses are produced.

The testing process is also a very useful way of getting ideas and opinions about how course theory can be applied to practice. Many trained nurses will recognise the difficulty of relating classroom taught theory to clinical practice. It might be believed that the commonly recognised 'theory/practice' gap would be even more applicable to open learning, but this is not so. Students who work through materials are asked to return all activities worked through, comments and notes, together with examples of schemes, records or other forms of documentation that they use as part of their own practice. This helps immensely in the design of professionally relevant materials. In 'Coronary Heart Disease; Reducing the risk' for example, it was possible to provide a range of real attitudes to preventive work, and some real opinions from health workers about their colleagues. This made teaching about teamwork more interesting, challenging and effective.

Relevance is also assessed by evaluation of courses while they are being offered. Those courses that are in the professional development area have as a stated goal the intention to change (improve) practice. Perhaps one of the reasons that the 'Nursing Process' course has been so widely studied is that it was found to do just that. In a study carried out amongst buyers of the pack in England the most significant finding to emerge was that use of the pack encouraged positive attitude changes.

- It makes nurses think about their practice and encourages change.
- It generates awareness of patient/nurse relationships and their influence on patient care.
- I am more aware of the total needs of individual patients and the accountability of nurses for patient care.

(Comments from nurses who have studied the pack.)

All courses follow the development process described above, whether they are to be at undergraduate, postgraduate or continuing education level. Many nurses are currently registered for courses at all levels of academic endeavour.

The undergraduate programme

The Open University offers a general degree which can be taken with or without honours and which is recognised as equivalent to a degree from any other British university. It is built up of individual courses which earn 'credits'. Six full credits (or equivalent) are needed for a Bachelor of Arts (BA) degree, and eight for a BA (Honours) degree.

Taking the equivalent of two full credit courses a year, the maximum allowed, a BA degree can be gained in three years and an Honours degree in four. However, most students progress at the rate of one credit (or equivalent) a year, to complete their BA degree in six years. This may not be as daunting as it sounds. Credit exemptions apply for a wide range of professional qualifications, provided they have been obtained at a higher education institution. The author of this chapter has a first degree from the Open University, towards which two credits exemptions were allowed; one for the Registered Nurse Tutor (RNT) qualification, the other for a Health Visitor's Certificate (HVCert). Being awarded exemptions usually involves students having to follow a special track. In the author's case this was education. There is still a great deal of subject choice whether one follows an open or a specialist track.

Undergraduate study normally begins with one or two foundation courses. These introduce the student to the university's teaching methods and to university level study, and provide a basis for more advanced courses in a variety of disciplines.

There are a wide variety of courses for students to choose from and some of the areas are indicated below:

— biology
— chemistry
— computing
— decision making
— economics
— education
— family and the community
— government and politics
— health and social welfare
— management
— philosophy and religious studies
— policy studies
— psychology
— sociology
— statistics
— women's studies

Research degrees

The research degree programme offers opportunities for advanced study and research leading to an original contribution to the published work in a particular field of scholarship. Students can work either using facilities in their home areas, with external supervisors appointed from local institutions of higher education, or full time at Walton Hall, Milton Keynes. Three research higher degrees are offered: a Bachelor of Philosophy (BPhil), a Master of Philosophy (MPhil) and a Doctor of Philosophy (PhD). They are awarded on examination of a thesis after the satisfactory completion of one, two or three years' study respectively: study may be spread over longer periods for part-time work.

The usual minimum entrance requirement for all research degrees is an upper second class honours degree of a British university or the Council for National Academic Awards (CNAA) relevant to the proposed research topic. Applications are also considered from those who, although lacking the normal entrance requirement, can show that they are appropriately prepared for postgraduate work in the proposed field of study.

Taught masters degrees

There are seven of these. Of particular interest to nurses will be the following.

- *Advanced Education and Social Research Methods* A two and a half year interdisciplinary course in research methods.
- *MA in Education* A modular degree which can build on undergraduate, associate student and diploma courses in education.
- *MA in Business Administration* This new course is offered from 1989.

Associate student courses

These include many of the courses available in the undergraduate and postgraduate programme and also a range of diplomas. Many of these courses are advanced. An Advanced Diploma may count as one third of the requirements of a taught MA. Students may register as associated students to follow a course of particular interest but disassociated from a degree course.

Of particular interest to nurses are post-basic professional diplomas. A professional diploma specifically links academic work with service provision and the development of skills. A professional diploma has the following characteristics:

— for the award students are required to complete the equivalent of two full credits
— the target audience includes people who are already experienced and who may already be qualified practitioners
— students are concerned not just with the acquisition of a body of knowledge but with its application to professional practice
— the focus is on the development of skills relevant to practitioners, and on the application of knowledge to solving problems faced by practitioners.

A number of professional diplomas (e.g. education, management) are already available and more are planned. These include a new 'Diploma in Health and Social Welfare' and a 'Diploma in Health Promotion'. Work has already begun on the latter.

Several courses in the associate student programme are popular with nurses. Many are in the fields of education and biological and behavioural sciences. Especially worth mentioning is a course offered by the Biology Faculty, 'Health and Disease'. This full credit course provides a detailed and systematic analysis of factors influencing health and disease in different cultures and contexts and explores basic methods of data analysis and application. It is also available in the undergraduate programme.

A course from Management Faculty, 'The Effective Manager', has proved so popular amongst staff that there is now to be a special remake using health service material. 'The Effective Health Manager' will be available from the end of 1989.

Short continuing education courses

However, the majority of nurses begin their open learning studies via continuing education studying packages produced by The Open University Department of Health and Social Welfare. This is not surprising, since it is the remit of this Department to provide for the education and training of health and health related professionals. As previously indicated, the Department does this by working in collaboration with key academics, agencies and policy makers in the health and social welfare fields.

Courses can be as short as 40 study hours in total, others are 100 or 200 study hours in total. Most courses are assessed and it is the Department's intention that in the future all courses will have an assessment built in. An assessment package is now being planned for 'A Systematic Approach to Nursing Care'.

A wide range of courses are on offer including:

Child Abuse and Neglect
Coronary Heart Disease; Reducing the Risk
Drug Use and Misuse
Mental Health Problems in Old Age
Caring for Older People
Caring For Children and Young People
Mental Handicap; Patterns For Living

Work going on for new courses includes a course on disabilities, another course on ageing, and new diplomas in health and social welfare and in health promotion. Work in these areas has arisen from curriculum work and research already going on in the department with the main areas of research being ageing, disability and the promotion of health. This latter area of work is one that is particularly important for nurses as nurses have been cited as being the natural leaders of the health promotion movement and will therefore have some responsibility for working towards 'Health For All By The Year

2000', a stated aim of the World Health Organisation to which the UK government is a signatory. Hand in hand with course development in health promotion is a major national research project funded by the Department of Health which is looking at the role of the nurse in health promotion work.

Summary

There are lots of opportunities for nurses to continue their education even if they cannot or choose not to do this by traditional methods such as college-based courses. Open learning also gives nurse managers and teachers the flexibility to support their staff development programmes as and how they wish.

Useful addresses

Council for National Academic
  Awards
334–354 Gray's Inn Road
London WC1X 8BP

For further information about undergraduate, associate student or higher degree programmes please write to the appropriate office (i.e. undergraduate if you wish to learn about a first degree) at:

The Open University
Walton Hall
Milton Keynes
Buckinghamshire MK7 6AN

If you wish to learn about programmes in health and social welfare please contact:

The Secretary
Department of Health and Social
  Welfare
The Open University (address as
  above)

Regional centres

With the wide range of courses and packs now available the amount of information that we are able to give here is very limited and you may feel there is insufficient detail for you to send for a prospectus and/or an application form. At each of the University's 13 regional centres there is an enquiry service. If you would like further information, please contact your nearest centre. The telephone numbers are as follows:

East Anglia
  (Cambridge)   0223 64721

East Midlands
  (Nottingham)   0602 473072

London
  01 7940575

North
  (Newcastle)   091 2841611

North West
  (Manchester)   061 8619823

Northern Ireland
  (Belfast)   0232 245025

Scotland
  (Edinburgh)   031 3324364

South East
  (East Grinstead)   0342 27821

South West
  (Bristol)   0272 299641

Southern
  (Oxford)   0865 730731

Wales
  (Cardiff)   0222 397911

West Midlands
  (Birmingham)   021 426 1661

Yorkshire
  (Leeds)   0532 444431

Maureen Eccleston
Head, School of Nursing and Health Studies
Stockport College of Further and Higher Education

4 Diploma in Nursing: Universities of London and Wales

The first level nurse, midwife, or health visitor is expected to provide a sensitive, individualised approach to the care of a patient or client, and to undertake a wide range of activities which require, amongst others, skills in collecting information, in analysing and making judgements about this information, and in planning and evaluating research-based care.

Also needed is the ability to manage resources effectively so that the care of an individual patient or client can be co-ordinated with that given to others. This developing clinical role is increasingly reliant on a sound theoretical knowledge, on problem-solving skills, and on the ability to respond effectively to changes and developments in health care.

Course details

The Diploma in Nursing is a course which has been specially designed to assist the nurse in developing these abilities, and to provide her with learning experiences which are highly relevant to her needs. The course has provided nurses with the opportunity to gain an advanced professional qualification of high repute for many years. It has responded to developments in nursing by adopting a new approach to learning, to ensure that holders of the Diploma are well equipped to meet their professional responsibilities.

A new curriculum was introduced at the beginning of the 1980s which reflected the need to move away from a medically orientated syllabus, with its acceptance of the traditional role of the nurse, replacing this with a health orientated programme which recognises the developing role of the nurse. In line with current educational thinking, the course emphasises a student-centred approach to learning and places great importance on the integration of theory with practice. As with other higher education courses, the Diploma is not so much concerned with imparting factual information as with helping students to understand the ideas and theories put forward by others and to develop their own thinking.

The length of the course is usually three years involving day release study, although one centre (Colchester) offers a two year course with other centres likely to follow suit in the near future. For those unable to attend regularly on a weekly basis, application can be made to study by distance learning thereby enabling students to study at a place and time which is convenient to them (see p. 4). Specially prepared learning materials are provided by the Distance Learning Centre which is located at South Bank Polytechnic, London. Tutorial support is provided by the colleges which have received approval as local study centres (the list of colleges is also available from The Distance Learning Centre, South Bank Polytechnic).

Whichever mode of study is decided upon, students will be expected to give some of their own time to their studies even when their employer is able to offer secondment.

Study requirements

Once enrolled on a day release course, the student will be expected to attend college for one day of each week of the academic year (this can be up to 36 weeks). Although the pattern of college terms may vary, there are usually breaks at Christmas and Easter, with possibly some short mid-term breaks as well. It is unwise to plan holidays so that they coincide with college terms as it may be difficult to keep studies up. If there is likely to be a major commitment such as a wedding to arrange, good planning will ensure that there are not two sets of deadlines to be met simultaneously. Illness is often less predictable, but as this too can interfere with studies, the course tutor should be informed immediately.

The study day may vary in length. Around six or seven hours is usual, although not all of this is likely to be spent at lectures as time will be allocated to individual study and to tutorials. Usually it is left to the individual student to decide how to use private study, although there may be occasions when students are given specific topics to explore.

Although at first many students feel anxious about their ability to organise their study time, this improves with practice. If particular problems are experienced, these should be discussed with the course tutor so that appropriate supporting actions can be taken to ensure that the student does not fall behind. Generally, the student should spend the amount of time equivalent to the length of the study day on their own studies. It may be necessary to experiment to find out the best way of doing this, particularly if working shifts vary from week to week. The aim should be to establish a regular routine.

Distance learning

If the student opts for the distance learning mode of study, the pattern of study is slightly different although the basic framework is the same.

The academic year consists of 38 study weeks and requires a minimum of 180 hours of formal study with additional reading time each week of around 8–10 hours. Ten per cent of the course is spent in face-to-face tuition at a local study centre where there is access to tutorial support and library facilities.

Although distance learning requires good organisation of time, many people have discovered that this method of study suits them very well.

Whichever mode of study is selected, a sense of commitment and the ability to motivate are useful qualities. One of the greatest sources of support in maintaining motivation comes from other students. Participation in study groups is encouraged as this provides valuable opportunities for getting to know the other students and for sharing ideas.

The outline of the course (London University)

Unit one   The human organism
The characteristics of living things
Differences between individuals
The individual and the group
The integrated functioning of the human organism
The behaviour of the individual

Unit two   Social organisation and social change
Organisation
Concept and nature of society

Social order
Patterns of change

Unit three   The application of care
Decision making
Concepts of nursing
Relating care to needs of the individual
Comparative systems of care

Unit four   Emergence of modern nursing and midwifery
The nursing role
The responsibility of the nurse
Preparation of the nurse
The nurse as a professional worker
Sociocultural influences on the role of the nurse
Comparative systems of nursing education

Unit five   Research and nursing
The place of nursing research
Research questions and problems
Ethical considerations
Statistics
Research methods

Unit six   Nursing
The search for excellence in nursing:
— special age groups
— special environments
— special forms of nursing practice

Two Units are studied concurrently in each year. The two year course covers similar ground but offers a more integrated approach.

In the first year, study of Units one and two enables the student to develop an understanding of the biological, behavioural, and social sciences which underpin health care and the practice of nursing. The course actively encourages the development of a clinical support system to enable the student to apply theory to practice.

Scheme of assessment

The scheme of assessment provides for either examination or assessment of course work. Whilst there is some variation in what is offered by individual centres, most students can expect to be assessed by course work with, possibly, a single examination. There may also be an oral examination.

Units one, two and four are assessed by either written examination or course work which comprises of three essays each of 2000–2500 words.

Unit three is assessed by course work consisting of two essays each of 2000–2500 words and a care plan. This is a detailed care plan for a patient/client nursed during the course of study for Unit three, accompanied by an essay of 1500–2000 words.

Unit five is assessed either by a written examination (one three-hour paper) or by course work. The written examination is divided into two parts; one testing knowledge of research methodology, the other testing insights gained into nursing by critical enquiry. If the student chooses to submit course work, two papers, each of 3000 words, must be presented. The first tests knowledge of research methodology in the form of a critical analysis of two published research reports from a short list and the other is based on a topic which will test insights gained into nursing by critical enquiry.

Unit six assessment is based on two papers which are prepared by the student during his/her studies for the unit. These papers are required to be original, unassisted, and based on topics of the student's own choice.

Each Unit has its own Board of Assessors headed by a Chief Assessor who, with the External Assessors, is appointed by Birkbeck College, University of London. (The course is located in Birkbeck College's Centre for Extra-Mural Studies at London University.) There is also an Internal Assessor for each Unit who is nominated by a centre and who is responsible for the Unit at that centre.

Although assessment can create anxiety for many students, it offers important benefits as detailed feedback is given on the course work to enable skills and understanding to be developed.

Also, as with any course, the assessment process provides a valuable means of promoting good standards. The Diploma is uniquely equipped to do this as it draws upon expertise from many centres of excellence in nursing throughout the United Kingdom. Clinical nurses, managers, researchers, and educationalists, who are often national and international leaders in their field, contribute to the development of the Diploma by acting as assessors, advisers, or teachers.

Entry requirements

The nurse must be registered with the United Kingdom Central Council for Nursing, Midwifery and Health Visiting (UKCC) as a first level nurse and hold a nursing post which either includes substantial clinical duties involving contact with patients/clients, or which permits the nurse to negotiate a suitable clinical commitment and to take regular responsibility for the planning and delivery of nursing care to patients/clients. He/she must also have attained a standard of general education which is approximately equivalent to that represented by the possession of a General Certificate of Secondary Education (GCSE) pass in at least five subjects, one of which must be English Language or Welsh.

If the nurse does not meet the educational entry requirement, he/she should consult the local course tutor, as it may be possible to assess his/her ability to benefit from the course by alternative methods. Although there is good evidence to show that adults without standard entry qualifications can do extremely well in university education, it requires considerable effort and perseverance. Probably the greatest hurdle to overcome is a lack of confidence. However, no-one should feel deterred from exploring the possibility of undertaking the course but, instead, seek advice on how best to prepare to undertake advanced level studies.

Preparation for entry

Nurses can gain more confidence and get back into a study routine by undertaking a course of study before applying for a place on a Diploma Course. The type of course will depend on individual needs. It is well worthwhile searching out a study skills course (see p. 8). These courses are now widely available either at local colleges or by distance learning (see p. 4).

Before applying to study for the Diploma, it is a good idea to find out what the course actually entails by discussing it with someone who has personal experience of completing the course. If at first this seems difficult, the course teacher may be able to help.

As good management of time is one of the most useful abilities to develop, any guidance on this is well worth having. Although advice on good management of time will be given by the course teacher, the more the student is prepared the better. Before applying to the course teacher of the local centre, it is a good idea for the nurse to discuss his/her plans with individuals who will be directly affected by them. If members of the family or friends understand from the beginning what the student is hoping to achieve, they are more likely to be supportive. They can also help in planning the best ways of balancing the nurse's various commitments, and may even volunteer to take over some of his/her responsibilities for the duration of the course. It is also important at this stage to decide which social or leisure activities are to be continued as they will provide valuable opportunities for relaxation.

Applying for a place on the course

At an early stage, the nurse should discuss his/her intentions with his/her nurse manager. There may be special secondment procedures which will have to be followed in order to apply for financial or other support. Such support entails the manager agreeing to second the nurse for the course of study. It indicates the manager's support for the student but readers are advised that there is a very wide variation in the levels of support given by employing authorities. Some employers have a fixed budget for the Diploma, whilst others have more flexible arrangements.

The rising demand for continuing education sometimes leads to a situation where the budget has to be spread very thinly, so that the nurse may find himself/herself being called upon to pay at least part of his/her fees.

Attendance requirements may also pose problems, particularly where there is a lot of interest in continuing education, as it may be difficult to release everyone who wishes to attend a course. The nurse may, therefore, find himself/herself being asked to contribute some of his/her off-duty time to his/her studies. Even if the nurse is not intending to apply for secondment, he/she should discuss his/her intentions with the nurse manager. The manager will be interested in knowing how the nurse envisages co-ordinating his/her studies with clinical or other responsibilities. Most nurse managers take the educational aspects of their role very seriously and are keen to give encouragement and support to their staff, so time should be taken to find out what support the manager can offer. The nurse should be prepared to explain why he/she wishes to apply for the course, and how it will fit in with his/her career plans. The manager will appreciate hearing these reasons and this initial discussion will help to prepare the nurse for the interview with the course tutor and, possibly, with a secondment panel as well.

No-one should be put off by the thought of interviews as they play an important role in helping the nurse to think carefully about all the implications at a very early stage. This ensures that problems are less likely to occur and the nurse will have the satisfaction of knowing that he/she has given careful thought to his/her ambitions.

Further opportunities

Once the nurse has been awarded the Diploma he/she will be thinking of what to do next! The enjoyment and the real sense of achievement experienced by students leads many of them to further studies.

Holders of the Diploma with a minimum profile of grades are eligible for admission to the once-calendar-year full-time course at King's College London, which leads to the award of the University's Bachelor of Science (BSc)(Honours) Degree in Nursing Studies. This Degree is now also available as a two year day release course at centres which offer the Diploma.

Diploma holders are also eligible to apply for admission to a number of part-time courses leading to the award of a Council for National Academic Awards (CNAA) Degree in Nursing and, increasingly, for a University degree course.

Many nurses report that promotion and new or interesting posts come their way after studying for the Diploma. Although, obviously, this cannot be guaranteed, the nursing service is always in need of nurses who can demonstrate an innovative approach to their work, who can manage change, and who can take responsibility for the active promotion of high standards of practice that are securely grounded in research.

The insider's view of the course

When asked about the course and its impact on them, nurses are enthusiastic about the Diploma in Nursing. One nurse said, "I really enjoyed coming to college every week and meeting the other students. We used to discuss all sorts of things, and I found it very helpful hearing what happens in other places. When you work in a specialised area you have no idea what is going on anywhere else." Another remarked, "I found it very hard work getting back to study again but I'm glad I made the effort." A student in her first term said, when asked how she was feeling about her studies, "I was looking after a patient the other day and all of a sudden I realised how much more I understood about what was happening to him. I felt so excited I rushed to tell the other nurses on the ward." Many nurses say, as did a student, "I have developed a lot more confidence in myself as a person. I can discuss things much more easily now with other people. They realise that I know what I am talking about and they take a lot more notice of what I think."

Any nurse who is responsible for some part of the clinical education of learner nurses will probably sympathise with the ward sister who gave as her reason for enrolling on the course, "All the learners were asking so many questions that I felt I had to make an effort to stay ahead of them. The Diploma has certainly helped me to do this. I no longer feel I'm running to keep up with the students when they come into this ward for their allocation." Another hard-pressed ward sister said with great feeling, "It was marvellous to have the day in college away from the ward as we are so busy there's hardly time to think. I feel the course gave me the opportunity to find out better ways of doing things so that the whole ward has benefited from me doing the course."

Getting started

If interested in this course, talk to the local course tutor or write to the University for information about centres which offer the Diploma in Nursing.

Useful addresses

Birkbeck College (*for the name and addresses of the nearest study centre*)
Centre for Extra-Mural Studies
University of London
26 Russell Square
London WC1E 7HU

Council for National Academic Awards
334–354 Gray's Inn Road
London WC1X 8BP

Distance Learning Centre
South Bank Polytechnic
Room 1D35
South Bank Technopark
90 London Road
London SE1 6LN

King's College London (*for
    information about the one-year
    degree course for holders of the
    Diploma*)
University of London
Chelsea Campus
552 King's Road
London SW10 OUA

United Kingdom Central Council
    for Nursing, Midwifery and
    Health Visiting
23 Portland Place
London W1N 3AF

University of London (*for
    information about the external
    two-year degree course*)
Secretary for External Students
Room 205
Senate House
Malet Street
London WC1E 7HU

Betty Kershaw
Project Leader/Director of Nurse Education
Stockport, Tameside and Glossop College of Nursing

5   Degree level studies

Despite the many opportunities now available for nurses to study degrees many still tend to shy away from higher education at a university or polytechnic. Many nurses, of course, have already obtained Open University degrees, while others are still studying with the Open University. This number will increase as the Open University develops the range of health care courses offered. A small but significant number are availing themselves of the opportunity offered by the Universities of London and Wales to convert their Diplomas in Nursing to degrees. Nowadays almost every university and polytechnic offers nurses the opportunity to study courses in higher education.

Through mature access criteria, any adult can apply to enter a university or polytechnic to study either full- or part-time courses. Each institute has its own selection process but all allow the applicant access to demonstrate their capability to study at this level through a variety of ways. Sometimes an applicant may be offered a place subject to completing a preliminary course which offers insight into returning to study as well as covering ground that an A level applicant would have covered during their college studies. Nurses usually decide to study part-time. Those who wish to undertake full-time degree studies, unless supported as tutor students by the National Boards, often find it difficult to obtain the necessary secondment even if they can arrange to have fees and out-of-pocket expenses met. Like all ratepayers or residents within a conurbation nurses are eligible to apply for Local Education Authority (LEA) grants as is any other applicant to university. Other funding may be available from the National Health Service Training Authority (NHSTA), the Department of Health, from Regional and District Health Authorities/Boards, and from charitable funding (such as the King's Fund). The scholarships which exist, as with Health Authority/Board funding, are very difficult to obtain.

A full list of scholarships available for degree and other studies can be obtained from the Royal College of Nursing (if the scholarship is needed for a nurse studying a nursing course). Usually the school of nursing and public libraries maintain lists and have specialist texts which list funding sources. Otherwise 'watch the nursing press' since most charitable and other funding bodies advertise their awards each year detailing who is eligible and how to apply.

As ever, a nurse seeking to study a full-time degree, just as with any course, should speak to his/her immediate manager. Secondment with or without salary support will need to be arranged, and the nurse needs to discuss possible Health Authority funding such as endowment or trust funds. It is advisable to find out as much as possible about the courses available before the nurse makes an appointment for such a discussion with his/her nurse manager. Whether full- or part-time study is wanted, information on courses available can be obtained from the university or polytechnic of choice. A more general leaflet PBD6/6/88 'Degree Courses for Registered Nurses' can be obtained from the English National Board (ENB) Careers Office, P.O. Box 356, Sheffield S8 0SJ. This gives details of courses available throughout the United Kingdom (UK), listing entry requirements, attendance regulations and the contact name and address. It is essential reading and is updated regularly. Also of use is the Health Services Careers Booklet, *Which Way?*, which contains more general advice and useful addresses. (This booklet is obtainable from Her Majesty's Stationery Office.) Before embarking on a course of any sort serious consideration to the work and time involved should obviously be given.

Full-time degree courses in the UK are invariably of three years' duration excluding any pre-degree studies the institute requires. Studying full-time is the quickest way to a degree; it is also the only way which will not conflict with the professional role of the nurse. An individual can then be a full-time student, concentrating solely on the course of study and not have to worry about what is happening back at work. However, most nurses, as has been said earlier, elect to undertake part-time study. Most employers will negotiate time off with an employee and many will be prepared to give some assistance with fees and travel. Agreed arrangements such as this are known as secondment. The nurse may be required by contract to stay with the employer for some time after completion. Completion can take several years, even claiming for credit for previous studies. For example, students holding the Diploma in Nursing of the Universities of London or Wales (a 3 year course) have to do only one year of part-time study to degree level, but those holding the Council for National

Academic Awards (CNAA) Diploma in Professional Studies in Nursing (a 2 year course) have a further two years to complete to gain their degree.

The University of Manchester and the Institute of Advanced Nursing Education at the Royal College of Nursing (RCN) offer a modular degree course. The nurse must complete ten modules, some compulsory, to achieve the degree; credit may be given for acceptable qualifications. The ten modules give a general degree, with a further three being required for honours.

Dundee College of Technology offer another route via certificate and diploma levels. Their four year part-time course also offers exemption for acceptable qualifications. The University of Ulster offers a three year part-time degree course which builds on their two year part-time (one year full-time) Diploma in Professional Development in Nursing.

There are many options available, and the only way to find the one which suits is to write for the ENB leaflet and to begin looking at what your institute of choice has to offer. Do not forget nurses are also welcome on part-time (and indeed full-time) degree level studies in many other relevant subjects; physiology, psychology, sociology, ethics. These are not given in any nursing list but should be obtainable from the nearest university or polytechnic. Write to the admissions office asking for details of part-time degrees in your area of choice.

Some courses, including those at Manchester and Coleraine for nurse teachers, incorporate two or three years' part-time study with a full-time year. The NHSTA has funding available to support certain courses which run in this way and, of course, the statutory bodies support their tutor students.

In the 1990s most nurses seeking higher degrees will be required to hold a first degree. Again, ENB leaflet PBD7/6/88 'Masters Degree Courses' is invaluable, listing a wide range of full- and part-time courses at this level. Provided the nurse has a first degree, usually honours, and usually a first or upper second class award, funding may be available from many other sources. The intending postgraduate would be well advised to discuss possible funding sources with his/her university or polytechnic tutor because as some course funding is specialised it may be allocated through departments rather than to individuals, or it may be restricted to students studying particular courses.

Masters degrees can be undertaken full- or part-time and are also available with the Open University.

The most common award is the Master of Science (MSc) or Master of Arts (MA) Method 1. Method 1 studies are examined and invariably include dissertation or thesis work. Method 2 studies are primarily research-based, but include some teaching often as part of a group. A Master of Philosophy (MPhil) degree is awarded for research.

Increasingly, research nurses are electing to undertake Doctor of Philosophy (PhD or DPhil) studies. This is the highest degree awarded and involves undertaking original research and presenting, for examination by viva, a thesis which is classed as source work – work which stretches the frontiers of knowledge. Applications for higher degrees need to be made to the university or polytechnic, taking advice from the tutors who supervised the first degree as concerns courses, funding possibilities and, if a research qualification, the various areas of study which may be relevant.

Summary

As the profession of nursing moves into the 1990s and Project 2000, more and more pre-registration students will be undertaking courses of preparation for the Register which award diploma and first degree qualifications. Increasingly the nurse practitioner who will work with these students will wish to undertake such studies themselves.

At the present time, all nurses have access to the Diploma in Nursing through either a local institute of higher education or with the Distance Learning Centre at South Bank Polytechnic. Distance learning is accessible to all. Degree level studies are available, as are diploma awards, with the Open University. These are increasingly health care orientated and more course units relevant to nursing are in preparation. More and more universities and polytechnics are offering nursing courses, and courses relevant to nurses, both full- and part-time. Sadly, there are areas of the country that do not have easy access to courses; it is even sadder when large conurbations do not have accessible programmes. For these nurses distance or open learning is the answer.

Degree level studies, through the Open University or the Bachelor of Science (BSc) (Honours) in Occupational Health at South Bank Polytechnic, are open to enrolled nurses, and they are as eligible to apply for places as is any other mature adult on other part- or full-time degree programmes. Enrolled nurses undertaking such courses must note however that the award of the degree does not award first level professional registration. Only a recognised conversion course can do this. However, there is no doubt, that an enrolled nurse requesting a place on a conversion course who holds a degree would be a most acceptable candidate for a course place. Nurses holding degree and diploma studies are valuable to the development of the profession and those who are training to enter it, and for the patients/clients with whom they work. The wide variety of choice available; length, full- or part-time, subject, and the many courses which credit previous learning, make degree and diploma studies much more accessible.

Write for the leaflets, contact your local institute, talk to your nurse manager and consider the options available. Find out about release, about secondment and about possible financial support. Choose the course which suits you best and stick with it. Many modules from one degree are credit-worthy for a degree elsewhere. After all, everyone has to move sometime. So, if you have started, do not give up if you have to move house. See what your previous studies can be credited with. Degree and diploma study does take time, but study can be infectious. For every student who gives up there is one who goes on to masters level and beyond. It must be worth it!

Useful addresses

British Association for Counselling
37a Sheep Street
Rugby
Warwickshire CV21 3BX

Council for National Academic
    Awards
334-354 Gray's Inn Road
London WC1X 8BP

Department of Health
Nursing Officer (Research)
Alexander Fleming House
Elephant and Castle
London SE1 6BY

Distance Learning Centre
South Bank Polytechnic
Room 1D35
South Bank Technopark
90 London Road
London SE1 6LN

Dundee College of Technology
Bell Street
Dundee DD1 1HG

Her Majesty's Stationery Office
49 High Holborn
London WC1V 6HB

Institute of Advanced Nursing
    Education
Royal College of Nursing
20 Cavendish Square
London W1M 0AB

King's Fund Centre
126 Albert Street
London NW1

National Health Service Training
  Authority
St Bartholomew's Court
18 Christmas Street
Bristol BS1 5BT

The Open University
Walton Hall
Milton Keynes
Buckinghamshire MK7 6AA

United Kingdom Central Council
  for Nursing, Midwifery and
  Health Visiting
23 Portland Place
London W1N 3AF

University of London
Department of Extra-Mural Studies
26 Russell Square
London WC1B 3DG

University of Manchester
Oxford Road
Manchester M13 9PL

University of Ulster
Coleraine BT52 1SA
Northern Ireland

University of Wales
Cathays Park
Cardiff CF1 3NS

National Boards

English National Board
Victory House
170 Tottenham Court Road
London W1A OHA

National Board for Scotland
22 Queen Street
Edinburgh EH2 1JX

Northern Ireland National Board
RAC House
79 Chichester Street
Belfast BT1 4JE

Welsh National Board
Floor 13
Pearl Assurance House
Greyfriars Road
Cardiff CF1 3AG

Every year each National Board publishes an index of circulars. This is available from directors of nurse education or equivalent post holders. The index gives details of all circulars, including those providing information on post-registration clinical courses, enrolled nurse conversion, and degree and diploma studies.

Stephen G. Wright
Consultant Nurse
Nursing Development Unit
Tameside General Hospital

6   A clinical career structure

For many decades, there have been very limited career opportunities for nurses who wished to remain 'at the bedside'. Beyond the ward sister/charge nurse role there were few, if any, rungs on the clinical ladder. Thus large numbers of nurses channelled their career advancement into two quite different directions; management and teaching. A third, nursing research, offered some very limited openings for nurses.

The opportunities for nurses in these roles to have clinical involvement (i.e. 'hands-on' patient care), let alone direct accountability for patient care, was and is very limited. The teachers and managers of nursing, for example, have less and less patient contact the higher up the hierarchy they go (see Fig. 1a). Presumably, other sources of job satisfaction take over, or perhaps these jobs offer an escape from the limitations and frustration of roles at clinical level.

In recent years, the opportunities which have opened up at clinical level could be described as an explosion (see Fig. 1b). The nurse job titles, however, might seem a little confusing. Indeed, anyone applying for jobs which seem to offer advanced clinical possibilities would do well to scrutinise the job descriptions very carefully. Precise details of the clinical input need to be thoroughly checked as well as examined during an informal visit or at an interview. Some jobs advertised as 'Clinical Nurse Specialist' for example, may well turn out to be teachers or managers by any other name.

However, with this reservation in mind, a very wide variety of roles now appear to be open to those nurses who wish to expand their activities and yet remain in clinical contact. Job titles such as 'Clinical Specialist', 'Consultant Nurse', 'Senior Primary Nurse', 'Lecturer/ Practitioner' or 'Senior Nurse' are now fairly common features in the nursing press. In addition, many managers have used the clinical grading structure imaginatively to expand the role (and salary!) of the sister/charge nurse. Sadly, in other areas clinical grading has not been

(a)

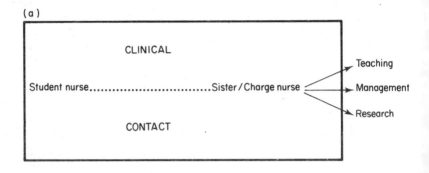

(b)

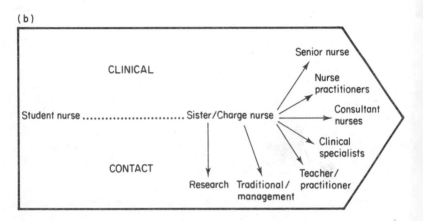

Fig. 6.1 Clinical career structures **(a)** The traditional model **(b)** The innovative model.

used in this way. Indeed, it has been used in quite the reverse – to restructure and reduce nursing costs. It will take some years before the principal aim of clinical grading – to enhance rewards for the 'bedside' nurse – can be assessed to see if it has become a reality.

The advanced clinical roles which have and are continuing to emerge for nurses, while they appear in many different fields, seem to expect certain prerequisites. However, as yet, there seems to be no national uniform agreement as to what constitutes a 'clinical nurse specialist' for example. Some job advertisements specify certain lengths of experience, postgraduate certificates, bachelors and masters degrees – others do not. Roles tend to be created and advertised on an *ad hoc* basis with very varying expectations of what makes up the suitable candidate. While this fluidity may be somewhat confusing, it does provide scope for nurses to expand roles in which they might not, strictly speaking, have qualifications or experience to 'fit the bill'.

Prerequisites to a clinical career path

There appears to be two main areas of interest. The features can briefly be summarised as follows.

- The background of the nurse
  - experience
  - degree of specialisation
  - specialist courses
  - postgraduate further education e.g. diplomas/degrees
  - advanced clinical skills
  - valuing clinical nursing
  - personal aspirations
- The opportunities available
  - management support
  - organisational structure
  - development opportunities
  - resources
  - management style and methods
  - local and national policies

The above are some of the key features which are affecting the development of a clinical career path for nurses and which will now be looked at in more detail.

The nurse's own output

While, to a large extent, advanced clinical roles depend on organisational factors for their development, there is a considerable amount that each individual nurse can do. This involves each nurse preparing himself or herself to expand and extend the knowledge and skills needed for further practice. It may also involve working within the organisation to assist in the development of new roles and the support of existing ones. In the first instance it requires a personal commitment for the nurse to keep up to date. This is not specific to advanced clinical roles (the United Kingdom Central Council for Nursing, Midwifery and Health Visiting (UKCC) Code of Conduct makes it a requirement of all nurses) but it does underline them. Keeping abreast of developments and knowledge can be done uniformly – by reading reputable nursing journals, research reports and textbooks, and making good use of local and nursing libraries. Also, by making the effort to seek out relevant courses, conferences and seminars or nursing open/distance learning programmes.

It is necessary to keep records of all courses of study (a new employer will want to have evidence that a nurse has kept up to date). It is also necessary to make decisions early in your career about which pattern you wish to follow. Nurses are increasingly required to become specialists in particular fields. Thus, some courses might be attractive because they are related to the nurses specialist subject (e.g. ENB courses in Intensive Care or Care of the Elderly Nursing). Other courses are more general in nature yet assist in the organisation of skills which can be applied in the specialist field (e.g. a teacher training or counselling course). It needs to be remembered that qualifications are of little relevance unless backed up with experience. Dore (1976) states 'diploma disease' is of little value to clinical nurses. Nurses need to be able to demonstrate an ability and commitment to apply theoretical knowledge. To this can be added the need for evidence of 'staying power' – not only in terms of the length of time in a particular job, but also the ability to complete a particular course of study. Also, it is worth remembering that more advanced clinical roles may require evidence of research skills and/or published research. New research opportunities for publishing should always be considered. Nurses are notorious for not talking about what they do or thinking it unworthy of broadcasting. Perhaps the first step for each nurse aspiring to a clinical career path is to accept that nursing practice is a rich and valuable entity in its own right. Each nurse can make a valuable contribution to nursing as a whole, as well as to their own career prospects, by considering opportunities to write about and publish their own nursing activities.

Setting objectives, therefore, forms part of the overall career plan that every nurse can make. It might be a question of thinking 'Where do I want to be in five years' time?' and then planning the steps needed to get there. Senior colleagues can help with advice and some nursing organisations designate specific nurses with careers counselling roles. The kind of job hoped for in the future will determine the necessary steps on the path towards it. For example, many clinical specialist roles require degree level education. 'G graded' ward sisters or charge nurses might be expected to do nursing degrees and/or provide evidence of further qualifications in management skills, specialist skills, counselling, teaching or primary nursing.

Deciding upon a career 'action plan' in this way can help many nurses toward their goal. Meanwhile, it might be necessary to examine the current area of practice for its possibilities. Learning how to develop 'change agent' skills might be an important aspect of personal development. These skills may be needed if the nurse prefers to remain with his/her existing employer where advancement opportunities are limited, but where the manager encourages the development of new roles by rethinking the old ones. Considerable skills are required to work within an organisation to produce innovation. Presenting a case, lobbying key people, arguing the facts, generating support – these and other skills are vital to any nurse who wants to introduce something new into an organisation. The alternatives are to accept the 'status quo' or to move on to a different setting where co-operation is possible.

Organisational commitment

Many nurses have shown themselves willing and able to develop clinical career pathways and advanced clinical roles in recent years through working in 'centres of excellence' such as the Nursing Development Units in Oxford and Tameside (Bamber *et al.*, 1989; Punton, 1989).

However, a nursing development unit is not a prerequisite for clinical development, as many nurses throughout the country have shown. Perhaps, the answer is that *every* place should be a nursing development unit – concentrating not just on developing nursing, but also *nurses*.

In response to development, some managers might be alarmed – We can't afford it'. The simple answer to that is 'We can't afford not to!'. Failure to develop nurses and nursing simultaneously contributes to the huge loss of nurses from nursing each year (Price-Waterhouse, 1988). The main components of an approach which appears successful can be summarised in the following way.

- Building up a programme of on site developmental opportunities (e.g. distance learning packs, on site library, journal club, seminars, workshops, lectures).
- Encouraging staff to attend off site development opportunities (e.g. courses and conferences).
- Identifying funding and time off arrangements and using these to the maximum, seeking alternative funding arrangements when resources are limited.
- Creating a support team of clinical specialists which provides
  — roles for other nurses to apply for
  — supporting clinical nurses in innovation and personal development
  — roles with direct input into practice.
- Setting objectives with staff, and providing career counselling, appraisal and performance review facilities.
- Forging links with schools of nursing and other educational establishments to expand the opportunities available.
- Supporting 'returning' of staff peer groups, nursing practice forums, group meetings, etc. taking place either at work (on site) or in a more social environment (off site).
- Ensuring that development opportunities are open to all gradings of staff.
- Organising care so that patient-centred practice is paramount (e.g. the development of primary nursing).
- Offering a flexible and creative management style which encourages research, experimentation and innovation in nursing.

For many nurses the examples cited above may seem hopelessly unrealistic and a 'pipe dream'. Others are fortunate to work in settings where such activities are the norm. Clinical nursing and the opportunities it offers is far more likely to prosper in such places. Those places in which the 'status quo' is preserved and in which no spirit of adventure prevails will ultimately lose out. They may, in the short term, contain costs and control the staff but, in the long term, they will find it increasingly difficult to recruit and retain nurses. Their ability to provide a service to the patient is then questionable.

In order to ensure that nurses are facilitated to maintain competence, the UKCC has set up a Post Registration Education and Practice Project (PREPP) which will identify standards of competence for the registered nurse. PREPP will consider the educational needs of all registered nurses, as these relate to maintaining competence, and will recommend how these levels of competence can be achieved through a structured programme of educational and practical progression. PREPP will include consultation with the profession and it is hoped, when developed, that it will assist in retaining well-qualified nurses in practice. Further information can be obtained from the Project Officer at the UKCC.

Developing a clinical career structure has been a slow and difficult process. It requires commitment and support for individual nurses and those in positions of authority in the organisation to pursue alternatives. Benner (1984) points out that becoming a clinical specialist is a long and difficult trajectory, but opportunities to put such experiences into practice, and yet remain with patients, do now appear to be expanding. The opportunity to develop must do, not only in the best interest of nurses and their career opportunities, but also in the interest of the service sector in which they work. Retaining well-educated, well-rewarded and well-motivated nurses at clinical level is something to which every patient has a right. Withdraw them and the high quality nursing service which the public increasingly demands will not become a reality.

Useful addresses

English National Board
Victory House
170 Tottenham Court Road
London W1P OHA

United Kingdom Central Council
  for Nursing, Midwifery and
  Health Visiting
23 Portland Place
London W1N 3AF

References

Bamber, T. *et al.* (1989). The Tameside experience. *Nursing Times*, 12(3), 26.

Benner, P. (1984). *From Novice to Expert*. Addison-Wesley, London.

Dore, K. (1976). *The Diploma Disease*. Allen and Unwin, London.

Price-Waterhouse (1988). *Nurse Retention and Recruitment*. Price-Waterhouse, London.

Punton, S. (1989). The Oxford experience. *Nursing Standard*, 22(3), 27–8.

Purdy, E. and Wright, S. (1988). If I were a rich nurse. *Nursing Times*, 84(41), 36–8.

Margaret Johnston
Tutor
Enrolled Nurse Developments
Oxford Health Authority

7 Enrolled nurse developments

The purpose of this chapter is to give an overview of the opportunities which have been made available within the last three years to help facilitate the professional development of enrolled nurses (EN) in Oxfordshire, so that this chapter can serve as a means to demonstrate what is possible. The overview is by no means exhaustive and is not intended to diminish in any way opportunities which were already available.

In Oxfordshire there are between 700 and 800 enrolled nurses working in general, mental illness, mental handicap, community and maternity services. Not all work full time but their development needs are similar.

The work enrolled nurses do is valued and changes which were occurring were as a result of changes in the way nursing care was being delivered rather than any failings on the part of the enrolled nurses. It was, however, recognised that opportunities should be provided to enable enrolled nurses to feel more confident and secure in their role and their position in the nursing team.

Even as far back as 1932, the Lancet Commission on Nursing talked about dangers to the public if a 'second grade' nurse might be entrusted, through ignorance of her limitations or for economic reasons, with responsibilities which he or she had not been trained to fulfil and disastrous results might ensue.

The United Kingdom Central Council for Nursing, Midwifery and Health Visiting (UKCC) Code of Professional Conduct (1984) refers to each registered nurse taking 'every reasonable opportunity to maintain and improve professional knowledge and competence'. It goes on to state that he/she should acknowledge any limitations of competence and refuse in such cases to accept delegated functions without first having received instruction in regard to these functions and having been assessed as competent.

In Oxfordshire, 1986, funding was obtained from the Monument

Trust for two years to support the activities of a tutor on behalf of enrolled nurses (other than for conversion courses). The Monument Trust provides financial support for innovative ventures. The overall aim of the two-year programme was to provide support and plan appropriate courses, and an experienced nurse teacher was appointed to carry out the work. It was successful, and after the two years' funding finished the post became a permanent one funded by the Health Authority. An initial survey carried out locally provided base line information which was useful for identifying major needs and planning. Work focused around three major areas namely:

— setting up of communication networks
— provision of 'support' and career advice
— meeting immediate educational needs

Attempts were made to improve communication networks, heighten awareness of current issues, and provide factual up-to-date information about changes taking place both locally and nationally.

Improved communication and a heightened awareness was achieved through:

— meetings to share information
— a newsletter 'Rollcall' which was printed quarterly and sent to every enrolled nurse in the District. Enrolled nurses were encouraged to help by contributing articles, making suggestions for improvement and distribution to designated geographical areas of work
— a radiopaging system was used by the tutor with opportunities for enrolled nurses to call her two set evenings per week until 10.00 p.m. thereby providing a service for those working unsocial hours
— the setting up of an enrolled nurse working group which met every two months helped practically in a number of ways and provided a 'welcome' service for enrolled nurses new to the district
— individual 'interviews' which took place as requested by enrolled nurses
— a large notice board especially for enrolled nurses which was constantly updated with current information, courses available, how to use libraries and information on open and distance learning; job vacancies were also put up weekly

Communication networks opened doors and provided new positive challenges. Despair gave way to hope and managers enthusiastically helped by participating in meetings, writing articles for the newsletter and allowing projects to be carried out in the workplaces so that enrolled nurses could appreciate the values of self-development and link these developments with reality.

Emphasis was placed on the fact that while the Health Authority was committed to helping all enrolled nurses develop professionally there would be no pressure to 'convert' to first level for those enrolled nurses who wished to remain as enrolled nurses.

It was recognised that enrolled nurses had been misused for years and now was the time for change. As one enrolled nurse said, 'By the time a solution is reached we will all be retired or dead!' Impatient enrolled nurses might be forgiven for thinking along the lines of Sir R. North when he said,

> A man has but one youth and considering the consequences of employing that well he has reason to think himself very rich, for that gone, all the wealth in the world will not purchase another.

While many complained of insufficient conversion courses it also became evident that many required a great deal of updating prior to successfully undertaking any period of intensive study, and good use could be made of the time spent waiting for a place on a course.

One of the reasons highlighted as to why enrolled nurses were dissatisfied focused around changes in work patterns and confusion over roles especially in the general field. Following extensive work involving the chief nursing officer, directors of nursing services and director of nurse education, a framework for a job description was compiled (Johnston and Ross, 1988). The position of the enrolled nurse as an associate nurse within the primary nursing setting was clarified (Manthey, 1980) and study days on the role of the associate nurse took place. Written philosophies and clear statements on roles and skill mix began emerging and these helped outline boundaries yet still allow flexibility within these boundaries.

Career advice was available for enrolled nurses and also for other grades of staff who might be involved in the management of enrolled nurses at work. This was linked with a personnel function not concerned with general administration of staff but seen rather as being concerned with people as individuals. The Institute of Personnel Management (1986) describe it as:

> The part of management concerned with people at work and with their relationship within an organisation. Its aim is to bring together and develop into an effective organisation the men and women who make up an enterprise enabling them to make their best contribution to its success.

Career advice centred around enabling enrolled nurses to obtain maximum benefit from performance reviews and other interviews with managers in view of the limited time which might be available to them. They were encouraged to develop a personal profile (i.e. a formative process of recording information which could be of assistance) (Garforth and Macintosh, 1987). The purpose of this was to guide them in a methodical way towards possible options for the future. Areas which enrolled nurses could explore initially included self-assessment – asking themselves questions like the following:

- What are my strengths and weaknesses, likes and dislikes?
- What are my educational attainments?
- What are my thoughts on my academic ability?
- Has learning theory been easy or difficult?
- Did I like academic courses or not?
- Was I a slow or fast learner?
- Did I enjoy learning in a group or alone?
- What do I know about open and distance learning?
- What are my thoughts on making use of open and distance learning?
- How have I coped with written examinations in the past?
- Am I good at work involving writing skills, using libraries, etc.?
- Have I thought about my ability/wish to travel and how far?
- What are my wishes for the future (realistic as well as idealistic)?
- Which new skills might I wish to develop? For example, many enrolled nurses working in mental handicap nursing have learned computer skills.
- What are my family and social commitments?
- What investment am I prepared to make for any self-development package both in terms of money and time (in some cases it might be worth exploring possible sources of funding for courses)?
- Where are the gaps in my clinical experience which possibly need exploration?
- Am I motivated to make a change?
- Do I know how to keep a curriculum vitae?

An overview of opportunities available would include encouraging the enrolled nurse to explore events in the local and national press, in libraries on notice boards, and to enquire about Health Authority courses, study days, courses organised by local schools, colleges of further education, polytechnic colleges, universities, open colleges, Open University, distance learning centres, careers advisory services, National Boards, professional bodies (e.g. The Royal College of Nursing (RCN)).

Self-development is encouraged and an enrolled nurse working in Oxfordshire has recently presented papers at two national conferences.

The aim of developing an enrolled nurse teacher was to provide an education which would be useful, cost-effective, marketable (i.e. it should meet the demand and should be worth releasing staff to attend). It should meet the needs of reality, be achievable, and not too complex. It would centre around the Oxfordshire Nursing Services philosophy of care which emphasises the value of expert nursing practitioners who can practice independently and be competent to meet all the needs of the individual patient. Learning should be viewed as a life-long habit rather than a series of 'one-offs'. It was hoped to provide new, exciting and varied ways of helping enrolled nurses update knowledge.

Courses which were developed over the two year period include the following.

- *52-week Registered General Nurse (RGN) conversion courses* which have been running since 1987. Work is underway to explore possibilities of including more flexible courses in the future.
- A *three day drug administration course* which runs regularly and is divided up into the following units of learning:

  — confidence and competence, legal and accountability issues
  — drug calculations
  — nursing precautions and responsibilities pre- and post-drug administration
  — consolidation of knowledge of statutory rules of drugs, for safe custody and storage
  — knowledge of specific drugs
  — patient education and motivation to take prescribed drugs correctly and reliably

- A *refresher/return to practice course*   There was a demand for this course to help enrolled nurses update and/or return to practice after a break in service. The courses have varied slightly, initially ranging from eight to twelve sessions (total 30 hours) with project work and supervised clinical practice in addition. Current courses span a six month period. Courses had previously been organised for first level nurses and these were extended to include enrolled nurses. The objectives of the courses were to provide experience which would enable participants to:

  — develop competencies which would assist them in the performance of nursing skills confidently, responsibly and safely

— understand and describe their professional and legal accountability
— demonstrate problem-solving techniques
— be aware and grow familar with new technology in nursing
   practice
— describe the importance of research and continuing nurse
   education

- *The use of distance and open learning*   Open University packages
  have been used extensively over the last three years and have
  proved especially useful for those working in isolation. Enrolled
  nurses have helped on two occasions with developmental testing of
  packs for the Distance Learning Centre at South Bank Polytechnic
  in London.
- Enrolled nurses are undertaking access courses prior to obtaining a
  place on a degree course.
- One enrolled nurse, frustrated by his inability to get a place on a
  conversion course, successfully found a place on a degree course
  (see p. 40).
- Study days have taken place on various topics such as days on
  finding out all about conversion courses and what is involved; the
  role of the associate nurse, the nursing process and improving
  specific study skills.
- Ventures already organised in the district were not repeated but
  extended where appropriate to include enrolled nurses.

Project developments

Simultaneous developments have taken place in the clinical area and
include the following.

Selection of bank/agency enrolled nurses

Bank or agency nurses no longer work in a 'protected' environment.
They are expected to operate in acute clinical settings, using current
approaches to nursing practice. They are used in times of staff
shortages and ward crisis and need to be adaptable, able to work
under stress, accept responsibility and be accountable for their own
practice, recognising limitations. In Oxfordshire it was recommended
that enrolled nurses were considered for bank work if they had

worked within the last three years in National Health Service (NHS) hospitals or a suitable equivalent. Those who had been away from nursing for some time might be required to undertake a 'back to nursing' course before being considered for employment. Concern was expressed about the wide circuit an enrolled nurse could be employed for and it was suggested that, ideally, they should be 'prepared for' and employed for one speciality or unit, for example medicine, surgery, paediatrics.

Regular study days were arranged for all 'bank' nurses and a number including enrolled nurses took advantage of the option to do the Open University package – 'A Systematic Approach to Nursing Care' (see Chapter 3).

Exchange schemes

Exchange schemes could benefit from further development. As an example of such a venture, an enrolled nurse working in an X-ray department in Banbury was able to visit an X-ray department in Oxford and spend the day with the enrolled nurse in charge of the department there. The enrolled nurses were able to exchange ideas and form links if wished.

Mental handicap services

A senior tutor in an education department and an enrolled nurse have set up a series of study days for enrolled nurses working in the mental handicap field. The Director of Nursing Services was particularly helpful enabling the enrolled nurse to carry out project work over a three month period, highlighting problems for enrolled nurses, and to be released on a weekly basis to set up study days and help to overcome some of the problems encountered.

Mental illness services

Night charge nurses have been extremely enthusiastic in encouraging their enrolled nurses to participate in development and have explored a number of ways to encourage self-development in addition to programmes already established. These included work on developing a learning package; 'adopting' enrolled nurses within their area of responsibility and setting up teaching programmes for them. Evening courses have been organised and have been well attended by very enthusiastic, hard-working enrolled nurses.

Mentor scheme

'Mentor' is defined by Longman as a wise and trusted advisor, (Longman Group Ltd, 1987). Experienced enrolled nurses acted as mentors for enrolled nurses on the return to practice course while undertaking supervised clinical experience.

A number of enrolled nurses with specific skills have taken on added responsibilities, for example trainers of staff on patient handling or teaching of specific skills, in X-ray departments or operating theatres.

There are numerous benefits for running courses for enrolled nurses from throughout the District, and from the different parts of the Register, but it has been equally important to visit different hospitals, community practices etc., and to hold local sessions/study days as appropriate. Some session/meetings have grown from requests from the enrolled nurses for regular meetings, and in Banbury the Director of Nursing (DNS) makes an effort to attend at least part of every meeting. These meetings have been extremely beneficial and are now developing into two-monthly meetings. From a general discussion the content has now developed and consists of lunch (optional), discussion about 'the topic of the day', a short meeting with the DNS, followed by an educational session.

There are many benefits derived from meeting as many enrolled nurses as possible, as frequently as possible, and this is partly achieved through running courses and attending meetings. Links are also established with the Enrolled Nurses' Advisory Committee of the RCN.

There are still many gaps in the service provided for enrolled nurses in Oxfordshire and it would be untrue to say that all enrolled nurses are happier with the situation as it is today. Many enrolled nurses have tried repeatedly, unsuccessfully for a place on a conversion course. If local enrolled nurses apply for a place and do not reach interview stage they have the option and indeed are encouraged to see the tutor to explore why and what could be done in the meantime. All those interviewed are told how they 'performed' and whether or not they are successful. It is not unusual for enrolled nurses to state that they have written over 50 letters to different schools in an attempt to secure a coveted place. At the other end of the scale there are those who have done little updating for many years and do not really see the need to change unless any training is mandatory to keep their job. They do not necessarily see updating as beneficial to their patients/ clients or themselves but rather as a necessary evil. As there has been some evidence of enrolled nurses being denied the opportunity to go on courses/study days in the past, some might be forgiven for displaying such negative attitudes.

Attitudes have changed considerably in students who have been fortunate enough to make the transition to registered general nurse (RGN) and one student who had documented feelings prior to and after the course was particularly honest about the change which had taken place. Many of those nurses could considerably influence enrolled nurses in a very positive way, pointing out the many benefits of making learning a life-long experience.

This chapter has briefly outlined some of the ventures which have been explored with enrolled nurses in Oxfordshire. Considerable influence on developments has come not only from enrolled nurses and other colleagues within the Health Authority but also from the many visitors, enquiries and letters which have all been greatly appreciated. It is recognised that many other Health Authorities are also doing a great deal to help enrolled nurses develop professionally and this chapter merely shares experiences gained in Oxfordshire and is not intended to be a perfect model. But every enrolled nurse has a right to know what his/her own Health Authority or Board provides and may wish to use the example of Oxford as a basis for discussion when learning needs are not as yet being met.

Useful addresses

Distance Learning Centre
South Bank Polytechnic
Room 1D35
South Bank Technopark
90 London Road
London SE1 6LN

Royal College of Nursing
20 Cavendish Square
London W1M OAB

The Open University
Walton Hall
Milton Keynes
Buckinghamshire MK7 6AA

United Kingdom Central Council
  for Nursing, Midwifery and
  Health Visiting
23 Portland Place
London W1N 3AF

References

Further Education Unit (1987). *Planning Staff Development: A Guide for Managers*. FEU, Yattendon.

Garforth, D. and Macintosh, H. (1987). *Profiling: A User's Manual*. Stanley Thornes, Cheltenham.

Johnston, M. *et al*. (1988). Drug giving for enrolled nurses. *Nursing Times*, 84(2), 13–19.

Johnston, M, and Ross, M. (1988). *The Way Forward. Clinical Development for Enrolled Nurses: A Guide for Managers*. Oxfordshire Health Authority, Oxford.

Longman Group Ltd (1987). *Longman Family Dictionary*. Chancellor Press, London.

Manthey, M. (1980). *The Practice of Primary Nursing*. Blackwell Scientific Publications Inc., Oxford.

The Dan Mason Nursing Research Committee (1962). *The Work, Responsibilities and Status of the Enrolled Nurse*. The Dan Mason Nursing Research Committee of the National Florence Nightingale Memorial Committee of Great Britain and Northern Ireland, London.

United Kingdom Central Council for Nursing, Midwifery and Health Visiting (1984). *Code of Professional Conduct for the Nurse, Midwife and Health Visitor*. UKCC, London.

Williams, G. (1982). *Learning the Law*. Stevens and Sons, London.

John Kelly
Regional Nurse Education and Development Adviser
North West Regional Health Authority

8 Management training and development

The recent history of management training for nurses arises from the recommendation of the Salmon Report of 1966. Since then considerable resources have been spent on providing nurses with a number of courses on management, often uni-disciplinary, and usually divided into three levels; first line, middle and senior management. This approach served only to compound the historical hierarchical structure of nursing and caused some discredit to the value of management training. There were other problems associated with this approach since many programmes were based on industrial models and used examples by a number of training agencies which were very difficult to translate into the Health Service.

Due to the volume of nurses requiring management training a large number of people were appointed to post without any form of preparation for their role and, subsequently, were often disillusioned by the seemingly inadequate management training and the inappropriate timing of their courses. Happily there has been a move away from this rather mechanistic approach, emphasised by the introduction of general management principles which focus on organisation. Within the National Health Service (NHS) the term 'management development' is usually accepted to mean a training programme designed to meet this particular objective.

There are a large variety of development programmes available at local, regional and national level for nurses and other staff groups which, if undertaken without some thought and preparation, can be confusing, time-wasting and expensive. Before embarking on any training programmes an individual, together with their senior manager, needs to identify the following key areas of learning.

- *Knowledge* What substantial knowledge does an individual need to know and understand? It might consist of various things such as:

— the environment in which a particular organisation operates
— the nature, function and role in an organisation
— theories of management

A note of caution: no one single theory of management is immediately available for individuals to resolve all their working relationships and difficulties.

- *Skills* This really is a catalogue of the various abilities any manager needs to have in order to be effective. Skills like planning, decision making, delegating, leading and influencing are all important and are often inter-related with qualities which are more personal such as judgement, creativity, mental agility, imagination and drive.
- *Attitudes and values* Possessing the knowledge and a wide range of skills is of little use if an individual does not understand and share the values of the organisation for which they are working. They will neither be motivated nor effective. It is very rare for any large organisation to actually set out in a formal way what its values are and thus develop a culture in which its employees can contribute. The NHS is not alone in this. In view of no values being available to you, a good starting base may be a concern for the consumer and a quality of care delivered. Independent health care organisations tend to determine these objections more clearly, and individual Health Authorities are beginning to do so (see Fig. 8.1).

From the above it will be seen that the task of management development cannot be discharged fully through the contents of an external course alone however high its quality. The process begins and ends at the workplace rather than in the classroom. This workplace to classroom gap must be bridged by focusing training on the practical problems of management faced in daily tasks, by making explicit the lengths between theory and practice, and by helping the manager to learn how to learn. Without this capacity to learn, experience fails to teach.

Within this working environment a key influence on the student, making for success or failure in the transfer of learning into improved managerial performance on the job, is undoubtedly that of the student's immediate superior, although senior management, colleagues and those holding second-in-line posts also have a significant impact. This calls for a far more positive participation in development training of junior managers and is normally found amongst the student's immediate superiors. It demands careful training and practice; a vital ingredient of any line manager's responsibility for the development of their staff. Ultimately, management, like much of

Purpose, vision and values

Stockport Health Authority is a large organisation by any standards. We make a vital contribution to the life of the local community as part of a wider network of health and welfare services. Everyone is affected by what we do.

It is important that we make a clear statement of what we are trying to achieve and how we intend to approach our various tasks. This leaflet gives a simple, straightforward statement of our purpose and the values we expect to see reflected in the way we all approach our work.

It is meant to guide our everyday actions and can help develop the strong sense of identity and common purpose necessary if we are to meet the needs of the people we serve.

Statement of purpose

Stockport Health Authority promotes good health, prevents illness and provides treatment and care services to the sick in order to improve the health of the community we serve. Our aim is to achieve this by effective use of our skills and resources in partnership with others providing and receiving services.

Statement of vision

We are committed to adopting the principles of *Health for All*. The key features of our approach to *Health for All* are:

▲ **Targeting health services to areas of greatest need.**

There are major inequalities in health between different social groups in Britain today. A recent report on the state of public health in Stockport confirms that this district is no exception.

Studies clearly show that the traditional distribution of health services is inversely related to need. For that reason, we need to re-examine services in Stockport and to target these at those areas of the community which have particularly high levels of social deprivation and ill-health.

▲ **Providing locally based health services.**

Most health care and education about health occurs informally within families and local communities. The role of the health service should be:

- to support the community in its caring and educational work
- to help people help themselves, their families and those around them to cope with illness, prevent health problems and promote good health.

Fig. 8.1 Purpose vision values.

To achieve this, our services need to be locally based, easily accessible and appropriate to local needs, while planning needs to be carried out in consultation with those who use our service.

The primary health care system provides the foundation for such a service and should be recognised and developed as the basis of the health care system.

▲ **Providing health services as an integral part of community services.**

Many factors have an impact on health. Housing, transport, education, leisure services and other things all affect our general state of health. We have an important role to play in putting health on the public agenda and ensuring that the health perspective is brought to all public policy decisions.

Health service workers must develop close working links with the local authority and the voluntary sector at every level so that we can provide a comprehensive and coherent network of community services – services which work together to protect and promote the health of the people of Stockport.

This is our purpose and vision – who and what we are and what we would like to achieve. Over the page is a statement of values, the ideas that we must apply to all our work to develop and improve both our services and ourselves.

Statement of values

▲ **To achieve the highest standard in the quality of our service, we must:**

- care passionately about the services we provide and work constantly to improve them
- value the individual
- treat patients as consumers
- provide a service that is both caring and proficient
- work towards excellence in the way we deal with people and in the technicalities of our work
- operate in partnership with other agencies, patients and the public
- provide equal health opportunities for all

▲ **Managers and staff can work better together if:**

- we all work in partnership, recognising the value of everybody's contribution
- equality of opportunity is provided and there is a high investment in the training and development of staff
- good communication and openness are practised at all levels in a working environment that is receptive to change
- innovation and responsible risk-taking are encouraged
- there is maximum devolution of responsibility to encourage and empower staff to do their best work
- we act with honesty and integrity, treating each other with trust and respect
- there is a clear commitment to action

clinical practice, is a practical art in which progress is made largely by constant appraised performance under the guidance of a trained practitioner. The model illustrated in Fig. 8.2 indicates a sequence of steps which are thought to be necessary if good practice and effective management development is to be achieved. This is presented within an overall management framework of staff development, and indicates that there are many means of developing staff other than through attendance at a management course.

As Individual Performance Review (IPR) becomes more established within the NHS, the approach to this kind of management development is likely to be extended.

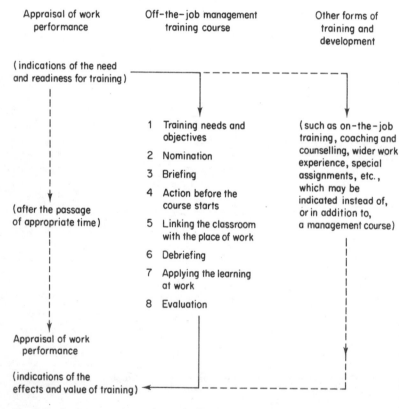

Fig. 8.2 Steps to good practice and effective management.

Courses available

Although some preparation for management is now included in the National Board's curricula for pre- and post-registration courses the majority of management opportunities arise elsewhere. The majority of Health Authorities Health Boards run some form of introductory management programmes for staff nurses/sisters. These may well be entirely in-house and of variable duration and content, whilst others may be linked with a more formal management qualification obtained in conjunction with a college of further education. A common core of these programmes would cover the following areas:
— management of patient care
— teaching and training in a clinical perspective
— ward management
— personnel management
— nursing research application
  A much more detailed synopsis of the content of these programmes is contained in the *Ward Sister Training Project* published by the Nursing Education Research Unit, Chelsea College, University of London (1984). Quite often these programmes are associated with the award of a Certificate in Management Studies provided by the Business and Technician Education Council (BTEC). Most nurses are concerned now particularly with the developments in further and higher education, and they should ensure any educational programme they attend is given the relevant academic credit. The Certificate in Management Studies and the relevant National Board courses fulfil this requirement.
  As nurses move into more senior management positions they often pursue further management education either at diploma or degree level and many of these can be undertaken on a part-time basis at the local university or polytechnic or through the Open University Business School. Your personnel department should be able to provide you with the relevant information regarding what is available locally. They should also be able to advise you on what support (if any) will be offered by your employer to undertake this further education. A list of management courses can be found in *The Directory of Continuing Education and Training for Nurses* published by Newpoint.

Management Education Syllabus and Open Learning Programme (MESOL)

The National Health Service Training Authority (NHSTA) has commissioned and developed a new foundation programme of management education for health service managers. This programme is designed to be a flexible, competency-based syllabus aimed at managers in the early stage of their career. It has been developed by a consortium of members of the Institute of Health Service Management and the Open University. The preparation of learning materials is now well advanced and is based on work already carried out by the Open University. The name of this programme is called Management Education Syllabus and Open Learning, usually abbreviated to MESOL. Although the use of open learning material has been available for a considerable amount of time, this is the first instance of it being targeted to a specific group of managers within the Health Care sector.

Pickup

The NHSTA has also recently commissioned a series of open learning modules described as health PICKUP (see p. 2). This is a total of 44 open learning modules which each take between 12–20 hours to complete. There are six initial modules available which have been piloted from September 1988, and they are as follows:
— The role of the professional in charge
— Setting objectives and standards of care
— Assessing needs and priorities
— Managing the caseload in time
— Helping staff learn to experience
— Working with other professionals

Health PICKUP is designed to provide flexible, modular programmes of non clinical post-basic training to qualified members of the nursing professions and the professions allied to medicine across England and Wales.

The training is skills-based and is derived from an extensive research programme carried out with the NHS. It is not intended to replace existing training initiatives but offers an additional resource to supplement and support existing activities. One advantage to this approach is that modules are designed to fit in with work and domestic schedules and they can be 'picked' to suit individual and/or service needs. This scheme is in its infancy and is therefore only likely to be available to a limited number of districts. Personnel departments appear to be running the scheme and the nurse would need to ask a district personnel officer for more information.

A further opportunity for nursing staff to progress within the management field of Health Care is via the NHS General Management Training Scheme (GMTS). There are three parts to this Scheme GMTS 1; GMTS 2; and GMTS 3. These programmes are co-ordinated by the Regional Health Authorities and further information and details can be obtained from them or the NHSTA.

GMTS 1 is designed as a first stage in developing a more suitably trained, high quality manager for the NHS of the future. It is open both to graduates with no NHS experience and to junior NHS staff who demonstrate a potential for general management. Inservice applicants should normally have little or no management experience or training and their current post will be unlikely to have much managerial content although their next post should be one at a junior management level. Successful applicants must be able to demonstrate that they have the ability to benefit from the experience available within the programme. Inservice applicants will have or in the near future expect to have completed their professional qualifications.

GMTS 2 is designed to meet the needs of more experienced managers in the NHS who demonstrate the potential for general management. It is probable that the experience of these managers will have been within the same discipline.

GMTS 3 is designed for senior managers preparing them for positions at a management board level.

These programmes are developed individually with practical placements supervised by a mentor who is usually a senior general manager. Incorporated within the programme is formal study usually at a university or business school. The number of nursing staff currently undertaking any of these programmes is extremely small compared with the number of nurses employed within the NHS. It may well be that individual nurses who have had some experience of management development programmes or a managerial post will now consider whether they would like to pursue this particular area.

Many nurses are confused between their professional development needs and the needs concerned with their current job and future employment training. Individuals will need to have access to sound advice and initially it might well be worthwhile discussing training needs with the personnel or training manager responsible for that individual's particular area of work. The decision as to which programme is undertaken will hopefully be decided by the nurse following discussion with his/her immediate manager by asking the questions outlined at the beginning of this chapter. However, managers may well be more likely to support nurses undertaking courses

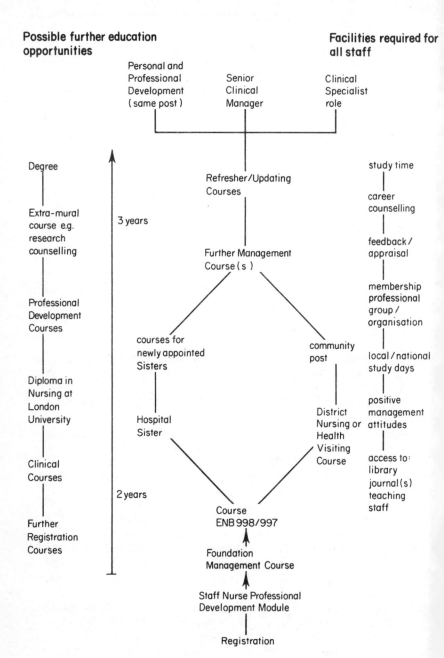

Possible further education opportunities

Facilities required for all staff

Personal and Professional Development (same post)

Senior Clinical Manager

Clinical Specialist role

Degree

Refresher/Updating Courses

study time

career counselling

Extra-mural course e.g. research counselling

3 years

feedback / appraisal

Further Management Course (s)

membership professional group / organisation

Professional Development Courses

courses for newly appointed Sisters

community post

local / national study days

Diploma in Nursing at London University

positive management attitudes

Clinical Courses

Hospital Sister

District Nursing or Health Visiting Course

2 years

access to: library journal(s) teaching staff

Further Registration Courses

Course ENB 998/997

Foundation Management Course

Staff Nurse Professional Development Module

Registration

Fig. 8.3 Educational requirements related to clinical career progression.

which are job specific (i.e. management and clinical courses) rather than those which enhance the professional role of the nurse (e.g. counselling courses, degree studies). This could be because managers are obliged to ensure that a nurse is competent to do his/her job. Increasingly, the enlightened manager is realising the value of professional as well as job development and it is always worthwhile discussing the issue. The model in Fig. 8.3 should be a better guide to where professional programmes (i.e. nursing programmes) intercept with management programmes and this provides a useful starting point for such discussions.

There is no doubt that nurses need structured management development linked with professional and clinical courses. The variety of options now available are beginning to bring such developments within the reach of all who need them.

Useful addresses

Nursing Education Research Unit
University of London
Chelsea Campus
552 King's Road
London SW10 OUA

The Open University
Walton Hall
Milton Keynes
Buckinghamshire MK7 6AA

National Health Service Training
   Authority
St Bartholomew's Court
18 Christmas Street
Bristol BS1 5BT

References

Lathlean, J. (1984). *Ward Sister Training Project*. Nursing Research Unit, University of London.
Salmon, B. (1966). *The Report of the Committee on Senior Nursing Staff Structure*. HMSO, London.
Wells, J. (1989). *The Directory of Continuing Education and Training for Nurses*. Newpoint, London.

Betty Kershaw
Project Leader/Director of Nurse Education
Stockport, Tameside and Glossop College of Nursing

9 Training to teach

The part the trained nurse plays in preventive health care is recognised in the United Kingdom Central Council for Nursing, Midwifery and Health Visiting (UKCC) Code of Professional Conduct (1984 and subsequent editions) and in the Competencies defined in the 1979 Nurses' Act. In order to best fulfil the demands this makes, it must be advisable for all nurses to develop some teaching skills. After all, we have all been taught by poor teachers in the past, and I doubt any of us learned very much. The nurse also has to teach other nurses, students, newly-appointed staff being orientated, auxiliary nurses, as well as para-medical colleagues, and, of course, the junior doctor. Having some skill and insight makes the job so much easier.

Developing teaching skills

The nurse seeking to develop teaching skills has a choice of learning opportunities available. In the first place the nurse should seek advice from the senior tutor responsible for continuing education to find out what facilities are provided locally. A visit to the library should produce a reading list which includes books and journal articles on all aspects of the subject. Inter-library loan may also be available if a particular text is not in stock and many libraries will obtain photo-copies of articles. It is usual to pay the cost of these services.

The department of continuing education should be able to provide information on teaching courses available either on site or at neighbouring institutions. These can range from one or two day courses helping the participant with a particular aspect of teaching, preparing teaching aids for example, to a course which has national recognition such as the English National Board (ENB) Course 998

'Teaching and Assessing in Clinical Practice'. There are many more opportunities to undertake courses to prepare the individual to teach nurses than there are to prepare nurses to teach patients, although with the commitment to 'Health For All by the Year 2000' we are seeing an increase in health promotion which can include short courses as well as relevant literature. At the initial stage in developing skills it is more important to take a course which is of personal interest. After all, the principles of teaching are very similar and it is not too difficult to transfer learning in one area to practice in another.

In order to teach nurses need to be able to communicate effectively at all levels. Explaining to a patient, client or family in 'simple terms' is recognised as totally inappropriate as the profession moves towards patient and family-centred care in which all are seen as equal partners. Most health authorities have communication workshops which allow the nurse the opportunity to explore all aspects of the art. Once the individual is confident that verbal and non-verbal skills are developed then is the time to move on to something more structured. Try to explore a variety of options, choosing the one that best meets your needs. Look at the courses which may be provided on site, and investigate what the local institutes of higher and further education have to offer (see p. 7). Do not forget the extra-mural department at the university which may hold weekend workshops. Do you want to start with developing your patient education or your nurse education skills? What you learn will be valuable across all aspects of teaching, but the workshop examples will be specific. As with every course, the cost of time and money needs consideration. It is important to ascertain whether or not the course has validation which gives credit recognition should the nurse wish to study further, or move from one post to another. For example, the Royal Marsden Hospital, London and Surrey, provides ENB course 998 on site. By an arrangement with a local approved institute, in their case North East Surrey College of Technology (NESCOT), the ENB course is recognised as a credit for the City and Guilds of London Institute's Further Education Teacher's Certificate (FETC) course (740), allowing staff to take the Institute course, with its wider national recognition, in a shorter period of time. There are many other schools and colleges of nursing which have the same or similar links.

Health Authorities that train nurses or midwives will almost certainly offer first level nurses access to the ENB 998 course or the parallel 997 course for midwives. Many also run short in-house courses to prepare all staff in training units for their role with students.

Alternative courses are available through the Distance Learning

Centre at South Bank Polytechnic as open learning (see p. 6). Two self-directed study units are published; 'Teaching Nurses' and 'Assessing Nurses'. Although these can be worked through alone it is of much more value to share your learning experience with a group of colleagues. Some continuing education departments will be able to assist by providing a tutor to lead the group. Some colleges of further education have nursing open learning publications in their Flexistudy centres (see p. 7), and may offer to mount a course centred on the material if enough nurses enrol to ensure cost-effectiveness. These courses may be linked to Business and Technician Education Council (BTEC) awards, giving national validation, and can also be offered for consideration for credit exemption for some ENB courses (ENB circular 88/67 RMHLV). Some schools of nursing include these study packages as part of ENB courses 998 and 997, which considerably reduces the time spent away from the clinical area, as well as increasing access for night and part-time staff.

Teaching skills are introduced in all National Board courses with the emphasis being consumer specific. The Diabetes Nursing course concentrates on teaching patients knowledge about their health problems so they can make the necessary adjustments to their life style as well as providing the nurse with information on skill training, in this case how to teach patients to safely give their own insulin. Should the nurse also be caring for cancer patients his/her ability to explain and assist patients and families will be readily transferable, as will his/her skill in teaching injection technique. Professional development courses tend to take a more global view to teaching skill training as does the National Board for Scotland's Diploma in Profesional Studies (see Chapter 2). Advice is offered on general approaches with the nurse being encouraged to pursue specific learning needs individually with tutor guidance.

The Distance Learning Centre at South Bank Polytechnic also produce a unit called 'Teaching Patients and Clients' which can be a most useful introduction for either individual nurses or small groups. The Royal Marsden patient education booklets can be helpful for those nurses caring for cancer patients, and organisations such as the British Diabetic Association publish their own leaflets.

Recordable teaching qualifications

The courses mentioned so far are primarily for nurses who wish to stay in direct patient care. For those who wish to expand their role to include a teaching remit other options are available. The health visitor can undertake a Field Work teaching qualification at his/her local institute of higher education, usually the one which offers Health Visitor Training. Similar courses are available for the Practical Work teaching qualification needed by district nurses. Provided the nurse manager supports his/her application, the nurse can expect assistance towards the costs from his/her employing authority, in return for a commitment to work for them on completion of the year's part-time course. The qualifications are recognised under the 1988 clinical grading review as attracting salary consideration and are recordable by the UKCC. Should further study follow, academic credit may be possible.

In Scotland the clinical nurse can undertake the Registered Clinical Nurse Teacher's (RCNT) course. Full details are available from the director of nurse education or the National Board, and expenses are met for those nurses who are accepted for National Board funding. As with all teaching courses funded by the National Boards, the nurse accepting Board funding has to agree to teach within the National Health Service (NHS) for a fixed period on completion (usually two years). There are no longer any RCNT courses elsewhere in the UK. Midwives who want to teach undertake the Advanced Diploma in Midwifery followed by the Midwife Teaching Diploma. Information about both courses, and the support available, can be obtained from the Senior Tutor in Midwifery. This course prepares the midwife for a teaching role in both patient care areas and in the classroom.

Nurses who wish to teach should also consult the senior manager, in this case the Director of Nurse Education (DNE) who will advise on the many and varied routes open to the nurse who is eligible to apply for support to do a course leading to the Registered Nurse Tutor (RNT) qualification. National Board circulars give the finite information on entry to courses: briefly summarised they state that the nurse must have a minimum of two years full-time (or the part-time equivalent) experience in a position of responsibility in an area where nurses are in training. He or she must hold an advanced nursing qualification, such as the Diploma in Nursing, a relevant degree or a long clinical nursing course (currently defined as those courses lasting at least six months). The DNE must sign a form stating that the person has the qualities necessary for teaching. Specialist courses are offered for district nurses and health visitors. Registered Sick Children' Nurses (RSCN), Registered Mental Nurses (RMN) and Registered Nurses for the Mental Handicapped (RNMH) take the same course as Registered General Nurses (RGN) but need to explore the options offered within specific programmes to ensure there is opportunity to develop skills or expertise in their area. Often specialist teachers in the school of nursing will be able to guide them appropriately.

Do not worry if you do not have the qualifications needed at first. Opportunity is available locally or by open or distance learning for the interested nurse to obtain qualifications. Often some support is available, and the prospective teacher should try to arrange to spend a short period in the school of nursing prior to commencing the teaching course. Choosing the course can be difficult. Some courses are now at degree level and, since the profession is committed to developing all graduate teachers as soon as possible, it is certainly worth considering these. Others offer the Certificate in Education (Cert. Ed) qualification with the opion for part-time study later to convert this to a degree. There are many different courses which allow a wide range of interests to be met and the best advice must be to go and see the senior nurse teacher, ask for the relevant National Board circulars, talk to newly qualified staff about the courses they did, discuss plans with the nurse manager, and then apply to the centres which are most appropriate. The nurse should consider whether he/she wants a full- or part-time course, whether he/she wants residence, and the nurse should also find out about the very generous support the Boards provide for their tutor students. You should be offered an interview: take it, and ask all the questions which still need answering.

Courses which are run in a university or within an institution affiliated to a university award their own certificates, diplomas and degrees which have national and international validation. Those run in polytechnics are validated by the Council for National Academic Awards (CNAA) and have the same level of validation recognition (see Chapters 4 and 5). Questions which need to be asked include those about crediting of the qualification when further academic study is undertaken, and about the opportunities that are available for further study. After all, it would be a waste of time re-doing course content which is what would have to be done if the course is not validated and credited. Once qualified, the nurse is expected to undertake a refresher course, at the National Board's expense, every five years. This is in addition to any updating done on the nurse's own initiative, or that which is otherwise provided.

Helping others learn is most rewarding, regardless of whether this is a patient learning to dress himself/herself after a stroke or an enrolled nurse passing a conversion course. It requires an interest in the person who is learning, in the subject being taught, and appropriate inter-personal skills. The best way to develop these requirements is within a group of people who share your interest. So find the course that is best for you at the time, and develop your skills from there.

Useful addresses

Council for National Academic
  Awards
344–345 Gray's Inn Road
London WC1X 8PT

Distance Learning Centre
South Bank Polytechnic
Room 1D35
South Bank Technopark
90 London Road
London SE1 6LN

English National Board
Victory House
170 Tottenham Court Road
London W1P OHA

United Kingdom Central Council
  for Nursing, Midwifery and
  Health Visiting
23 Portland Place
London W1N 3AF

Betty Kershaw
Project Leader/Director of Nurse Education
and
Mary Harrison
Librarian
Stockport, Tameside and Glossop College of Nursing

10   What your Health Authority has to offer

Inservice training

Although many Health Authorities now incorporate traditional inservice training with professional continuing education there are nurses who do not have the opportunity to benefit from this co-ordinated approach. An active inservice training department can help such nurses by providing relevant and applicable professional development. The staff in such departments need to work very closely with nurse managers to ensure local learning objectives are met.

Often a new member of staff is introduced to the department through orientation or induction programmes (see p. 56). Sometimes this consists of a planned course with other staff new to the Health Authority, or it takes the form of an individual programme planned to meet very specific objectives. Increasingly a combination of techniques is used, with clinical staff being given some practical induction as well.

In an inservice training department the teaching staff will respond to a wide variety of requests for updating, often updating that is relevant to non-nurses as well. They are frequently charged with providing necessary review sessions on health and safety issues such as fire training, resuscitation, and safe lifting techniques. Most Health Authorities require staff to update in these areas at least annually. Inservice trainers may also be expected to ensure 'new' policies and practices are introduced to the staff involved. The 1983/84 change to U100 insulin was brought to the attention of staff largely through inservice training, and the more recent information on AIDS and salmonella hazards has often been disseminated in a similar way. So, nurses seeking updating on or new knowledge about their own

Authority's policies and practices would be well advised to approach the inservice training officer. Most courses can be offered to staff outside the health authority if there is an identified need. A fee is usually charged for this service.

The department is also expected to mount courses at management's request. Where authorities are using Individual Performance Review (IPR) as a means of analysing staff development needs, this information can be collated and used to direct inservice training provision. It may be that the first identified need is for an introductory programme for managers on IPR! Other topics could include ward budgeting, team leadership, developing interview skills, all of which are competencies needed by clinical staff.

Management may also request individual or group programmes for staff who are changing jobs. As patients in mental health and mental handicap units are moved into the community, staff need to learn new skills. Some key staff will obviously attend National Board courses but most, including auxiliary nurses, will need development on site. Sometimes when there has been a problem in a unit, for example with the storage and administration of drugs, managers will request remedial teaching again for an individual or group.

The good inservice trainer will also respond to requests from staff at the grass roots. After all, it is these nurses who are in day-to-day contact with the patients and who are best able to identify what they need in order to care better. One way to reach this group is through a questionnaire; another by course follow-up and evaluation.

In smaller, and non-training hospitals, it is this inservice training department which is becoming involved with back to nursing courses and support worker (health care assistant) development. They may run 'Keep-in-Touch' clubs, organise study days and conferences for nurses from both within and from outside the Health Authority, and often have a remit which includes other staff groups.

The experienced inservice training officer is a major source of information to nursing staff. Because of close links with non-nurse training and thus with personnel departments, the inservice training officer can offer guidance on, for example, courses such as the Certificate and Diploma in Management and about funding available within the Authority for staff who wish to undertake these and other externally managed courses. For management training at an advanced level it may be appropriate to seek out the personnel officer, just as the clinical nurse who wanted information on reverse barrier nursing would seek out the infection control officer. Departmental staff can advise on the location of such people.

Contrary to expectations, all inservice training courses do not involve sitting in classrooms. There are many educational programmes, such as those with the Open University and the Distance Learning Centres, which the department staff can advise about and facilitate access. Often they co-ordinate information on external courses and conferences, and can guide the enquiring nurse who is seeking specialist help. Visits to centres of excellence to gain insight into a new idea for practice can often be facilitated, as can clinical updating when a new idea or piece of equipment is to be introduced into a clinical setting. The good department can act as the focal point for trained staff development and, together with the trained librarian, go a long way to helping staff meet identified learning needs.

The skilled librarian, although not a part of the inservice training department, is integral in helping staff meet their full potential, and the facilities offered are invariably available to all staff.

Using libraries

Libraries are an indispensable resource for the nurse interested in keeping up to date. The first step is to find out what library resources are available locally, beginning with the public library. If difficulties are experienced in learning about additional library resources, consult the list of regional librarians willing to offer advice published in the *Nursing Standard* on 24 September 1988.

Britain has one of the world's greatest public library networks, offering an extensive range of information services at minimal cost. In addition, many university, polytechnic and college libraries are open to non-students, although services may be restricted and a membership fee may be imposed.

Within the hospital environment, most schools of nursing and postgraduate medical centres operate libraries. In many cases, these are open not only to tutorial staff and students, but also to trained staff. The size and scope of these special libraries varies greatly from region to region, depending upon the funding allocated and the importance given to the library's role in education. Increasingly, such libraries are seen as fundamental to the provision of education and are well-stocked with the latest available journals, books and other information sources. They are staffed by qualified professional librarians, whose training and expertise enable them to offer the best in library service.

In addition, there are other special libraries available to the enquiring researcher. All members of the Royal College of Nursing (RCN) are entitled to use the RCN's library services. These include provision of photocopies of journal articles at a reasonable cost, lending of up to four books at a time, provided the borrower absorbs any postal charges, and free literature searches of the computerized version of the RCN's *Nursing Bibliography*. Members of the Royal College of Midwives (RCM) are able to use the RCM Library, also in London. A list of additional health libraries, plus a description of their accessibility and services, can also be found in the *Nursing Standard* of 24 September, 1988.

It is recommended that readers approach thier local libraries first and contact the more specialised and distant libraries only if local resources fail to meet their needs.

When first using a library, many people experience some apprehension about approaching library staff and asking for assistance. A common fear, but one which must be overcome in order to make efficient use of a library's resources. Although all libraries adhere to certain basic organisational principles, each library has its own individual characteristics and peculiarities. The first-time visitor to any library is strongly recommended to ask at the information desk for a tour of the library's facilities and an explanation of its services. Never be afraid of showing a lack of knowledge about how to use a library or its resources. Library staff will not interpret this as ignorance or stupidity; rather, they will see it as a sign of a serious researcher.

In order to facilitate the use of their book collections, libraries prepare catalogues, which are basically lists of the books contained in the collection. Three formats are common: the traditional card catalogue; microfiche; and the computerised catalogue. Whatever the format, the catalogue will offer access to the library collection, most commonly by author, title of the book, and subject. Information on the catalogue record will direct the reader to the area of the library in which the desired book is shelved. As cataloguing systems vary from library to library, it is recommended that the reader always ask for an explanation of the catalogue arrangement and use.

Correct use of the catalogue will save the reader time and will offer a complete picture of the contents of the library. If a desired book is not on the shelf, it is most likely on loan. Most libraries will reserve such books and notify requesting readers when they are returned. A small fee is often charged for this service.

The library journal collection has two potential uses. Setting aside a specific time each week to look at the most recent issues of nursing journals will enable the practising nurse to keep abreast of developments in the profession. In addition, journals are an important resource when material on a specific subject is desired; they tend to be more current and concise than most books.

In order to locate articles on a particular subject, the use of periodical indexes is recommended. These are lists of journal articles, arranged by subject and published on a regular basis. Of particular interest to the professional nurse will be the RCN's *Nursing Bibliography*, which lists articles published in over 200 nursing journals, both British and international. The accompanying annual list of subject headings should be consulted at the start of any literature search in order to establish the correct subject heading to use.

Other potentially useful indexes include the Department of Health's (previously the DHSS) library publications, *Nursing Research Abstracts* and *Health Service Abstracts* and the American publications, *Cumulative Index to Nursing and Allied Health Literature* and *International Nursing Index*. Again, before starting the literature search, refer to the subject indexes in order to establish the appropriate terms to use.

Many periodical indexes are now available in a computerised format which enables professional librarians to prepare special subject bibliographies more efficiently and quickly than is possible using the printed versions. Find out if your library offers an on-line search service. In most cases, there will be a cost involved. This will vary depending on such factors as the databases used, the time required to do the search, and the number of bibliographic references needed. Usually the librarian will do the actual searching, following an interview in which the specific needs of the reader are identified.

Should the reader require books or journal articles which are not in the library collection, an interlibrary loan may be possible. Public libraries and many smaller libraries offer this service, which involves borrowing the book or obtaining a photocopy of the article from another library. This can take time and sometimes involves a fee charged to the reader.

If for some reason a library fails to satisfy your requirements, point this out politely to the library staff. Perhaps your information request has been misunderstood. Or perhaps there is a gap in the collection which your comments will identify. Librarians, always interested in meeting the information needs of readers, welcome suggestions.

There is a wealth of published information available in Britain's libraries. It is there to be used, and library staff are there to help you to use it.

Libraries open to Health Authority staff

It is advisable to write to check opening times and readership requirements (some libraries require letters of recommendation).

The Department of Health
Alexander Fleming House
The Elephant and Castle
London   SE1 6BY

Tel. 01–407 5522

The Health Promotional
   Information Service
Health Education Authority
78 New Oxford Street
London   WC1A 1AH

Tel. 01–631 0930

The Health Visitor's Association
50 Southwark Street
London   SE1 1UN

Tel. 01–378 7255

The King's Fund Centre
126 Albert Street
London   NW1 7NF

Tel. 01–267 6111

The King's Fund College
2 Palace Court
London   W2 4HS

Tel. 01-727 0581

Northern Ireland Health and Social
   Services Library
Queen's University
Institute of Clinical Services
Grosvenor Road
Belfast   BT12 6BJ

Tel. 0232–322043

The Royal College of Midwives
15 Mansfield Street
London   W1M 0BE

Tel. 01–580 6523

The Royal College of Nursing
20 Cavendish Square
London   W1M 0AB

Tel. 01–409 3333

Scottish Health Service Library
Crewe Road South
Edinburgh   EH4 3LF

Tel. 031–332 2335

The University of Wales
School of Medicine
Heath Park
Cardiff   CF4 4XN

Tel. 0222–755944

Wellcome Institute for the History
   of Medicine
183 Euston Road
London   NW1 2BP

Tel. 01–387 4477

Useful addresses

Distance Learning Centre
South Bank Polytechnic
Room 1D35
South Bank Technopark
90 London Road
London SE1 6LN

The Open University
Walton Hall
Milton Keynes
Buckinghamshire MK7 6AA

References

Editorial (1988).   With reference to. *Nursing Standard*, **2(51)**, 20–1.

Stephen G. Wright
Consultant Nurse
Nursing Development Unit
Tameside General Hospital

11 Making changes

It is difficult to attend any meeting today, switch on the television or read a book without coming across the notion that 'things are changing!' 'We are all in the business of change' states Toffler (1973), who also argues that we cannot avoid change, for it is accelerating and we are all being swept along with it. Nursing is no exception to this, for it has seen monumental changes in the relatively few years since Florence Nightingale burst upon the scene and it has even greater challenges ahead.

Many of the aspects of this book have been about change; the need for the organisation to adapt to changes, and for the nurse to re-examine his or her own role and direction.

Changing things, however, is a risky activity. 'Sometimes it is safer to be in chains than to be free' wrote Kafka (1916). Perhaps it would be 'safer' if nurses kept themselves in their place, and did as the doctors said, and avoided disturbing the status quo. 'No change', however, does not appear to be an option for nurses, for change is directed at us from many different directions – patients' expectations, our own aspirations, new government policies, changing health demands and so on. Nurses will have to change, we have no choice. However, there are risks in change, how can these be minimised?

Entering the process of change unprepared, unplanned and without the skills of being a change agent is not unlike walking naked and defenceless into the jungle. Two key areas need to be considered if nurses are not to come to harm in the change process. Firstly, the nurse needs to develop knowledge and skill as a change agent and, secondly, an awareness of how the organisation and the people in it function.

It is not possible, within the confines of this chapter, to explore these issues in greater detail. More and more texts are now emerging, written by nurses and often based on considerable experience, describing how nurses can work successfully as change agents

(Wright, 1989; Clay, 1987; Campbell, 1984 and Pearson, 1985). However, a few crucial issues can be discussed here.

The hero-innovator

Often in nursing a bright, enthusiastic person is put in post when a problem arises in a unit and asked to solve it. They often throw themselves with great energy into the task, only to end up burned out and defeated. Any changes made are superficial and soon reversed. Indeed using the 'myth of the hero-innovator' (Georgiades, 1975) might be a tool to prevent change lasting. If the change process collapses the change agent moves on; if it fails while they are still active, then it can be excused as 'unworkable' anyway. Meanwhile, management was at least perceived as trying to do something. Nurses need to be very wary of being drawn into such roles and having their energies abused in this way.

Resistance

Resistance to change is the greatest obstacle for the change agent to overcome. It can arise from all quarters and can be so powerful as to subvert and completely defeat any proposed changes. It is also worth remembering that not all changes are necessarily improvement – sometimes resisting change is a positive activity and not always a negative one (e.g. resisting privatisation of health care might be viewed as either 'good' or 'bad' depending on the nurse's personal perspective).

Rogers (1962) has shown that the desire for change can come from a very small percentage (less than two per cent) within an organisation while large numbers will be more sceptical, if ultimately compliant. Even so, resistance from a sizeable majority of 'laggards' (about 15–20 per cent) can be expected and sustained for long periods. The cost, in conflict and exhaustion for both the change agent and all concerned, can be enormous. In nursing, there can be even greater costs – for the vulnerable client or patient caught in the middle of it.

The need for a change strategy

Various methods of changing nursing are on offer; but some appear to be less applicable to nursing than others (Wright, 1989).

The power–coercive method ,

The power–coercive method tells people what to do (e.g. 'you will do the nursing process', 'you will organise your ward in this way'). This 'telling' approach, it is argued, is inappropriate where long-term change is needed. It may last for a little while when the 'teller' is present, but when he/she disappears the nurses and the changes revert to what they were before. (As soon as the sister/charge nurse goes off duty, the staff do things the way they always did!)

The rational–empirical method

The rational–empirical method assumes that people will respond in a logical way when given the evidence (e.g. research shows something to be wrong in nursing, therefore all nurses will change their behaviour accordingly). It assumes, for example, that the smoker will give up smoking when faced with the facts of the ill-health it causes.

The normative–re-educative method

The normative–re-educative method seeks to get groups of nursing staff together to help solve their problems and make changes. It is this method, particularly when combined with the support of a skilled and knowledgeable change agent, which appears to be most effective in producing long-term change to new ways of doing things (Wright, 1989; Pearson, 1985 and Ottoway 1976 and 1980). By ensuring that the staff own the changes they have made, and by raising their awareness of what needs to be and can be changed, then it seems possible to effect real change in nursing. The change agent introduces new ideas in a non-authoritarian way, but also by working as a partner with colleagues to generate innovation and promote new norms.

Planning the change

This involves an almost 'nursing process' type approach such as assessing what needs to be changed, the circumstances which will help the change process, planning the approach, carrying it through and then evaluating the success. While a planned approach is strongly advocated by Pearson and Vaughan (1986), a considerable degree of flexibility and adaptability is needed, particularly in the part of the change agent (Wright, 1989). Change is rarely so linear and straight-forward and requires considerable skill in pursuing it. It takes considerable time and effort and requires a 'mapping out' of the environment so that conflicts can be minimised and obstacles overcome. Managers and teachers have a particularly important role to play in assisting and supporting the change agent and the clinical staff who are introducing clinical innovations. Failing in these quarters will at best delay, at worst obstruct, any possible changes.

Becoming a change agent

In some respects, all nurses are change agents. The day-to-day work they do with patients and clients involves helping them to make changes in their lives. The skills needed influence not just their ability to change, but their ability to help patients. These skills include:

— knowledge and awareness of nursing; the organisation and individual behaviour
— communication and interpersonal skills
— self-awareness and assertiveness
— physical and psychological stamina
— knowledge, awareness and skill in change strategies and processes
— ability to work with groups, colleagues and those in authority

Many nurses acquire these and other skills intuitively. But most nurses need a planned approach to help them acquire the skills of change agency as part of their (lifelong) education in nursing. Unfortunately, the type of courses on offer to nurses contain few, if any, of the above elements. Becoming a change agent requires that nurses seek development in the appropriate skills outside their usual place of employment. Perhaps this lack of attention to change agency skills in traditional nurse education is not surprising. After all, it might 'rock the boat' too much. There are at least half a million nurses in the

United Kingdom. I can imagine what effect hundreds of thousands of skilled, assertive and aware change agent nurses would have, not just on nursing, or even health care, but on society as a whole! Perhaps some might think it better if nurses were kept quietly in their place!

Making changes can be immensely difficult. It is fraught with conflict and dangers for nurses and their colleagues. The opportunity for nurses to change things is intimately bound up with the opportunity to develop as change agents. Because of the nature of nursing this is particularly related to the roles of nurses and the way they develop, not just in nursing but in society in the wider sense. Becoming a knowledgeable and skilful change agent will minimise conflicts and enhance the changes of success. The reader who would change things is urged to pursue such knowledge and skills in greater depth before setting out on the road of change.

This book has been all about maintaining professional competence and expanding both nurses and nursing horizons. There are limits to how much of this can be done alone. There are dangers in trying to force new knowledge and ideas upon colleagues or on the organisation. However important and logical the new aspect which each nurse learns as they develop might be, this chapter has suggested that large numbers of colleagues might be less than enthusiastic about taking the new ideas on board. It is one thing to know what needs changing, quite another to know how to change.

To some degree, each nurse can learn to be a change agent and pass their skills to colleagues. Raising the consciousness of nurses as to what nursing is, and what it might be, is the first step in the direction of long-term change. Thus equipped, nurses are better able to improve the quality of life for themselves, and also those patients whom they exist to serve.

References

Campbell, A.V. (1984). *Moderated Love*. SPCK, London.
Clay, T. (1987). *Nurses, Power and Politics*. Heinemann, London.
Georgiades, N.J. and Phillimore, L. (1975). The myth of the hero-innovator. *In* Kiernan, C.C. and Woodford, F.B. (Eds) *Behaviour Modification with the Severely Retarded*. Associated Scientific Publications, London.
Kafka, F. (1916). *Metamorphosis*. Penguin, Harmondsworth.
Ottoway, R.N. (1976). A change strategy to implement new norms,

new styles and new environment in the work organisation. *Personnel Review*, 5(1), 13–18.

Ottoway, R.N. (1980). *Defining the Change Agent*. Unpublished paper. Department of Management Sciences, University of Manchester Institute of Technology.

Pearson, A. (1985). *The Effects of Introducing New Norms in a Nursing Unit*. Unpublished PhD Thesis, Goldsmith's College, University of London.

Pearson A. and Vaughan, B. (1986). *Nursing Models for Practice*. Heinemann, London.

Rogers, E.M. (1962). *Diffusion of Innovations*. Free Press, New York.

Toffler, A. (1973). *Future Shock*. Pan Books, London.

Wright, S.G. (1989). *Changing Nursing Practice*. Edward Arnold, Kent.

Index